What the Fat?

What the Fat?

How to live the ultimate
Low-Carb, HEALTHY-*Fat* lifestyle

THE PROFESSOR	THE DIETITIAN	THE CHEF
Grant Schofield	Dr. Caryn Zinn	Craig Rodger

Foreword Nina Teicholz | *Introduction* Pete Evans

weldon**owen**

To Caryn Zinn's precious mother, Denise,
who sadly lost her battle with cancer on
5 April 2015. She is dearly missed.

Contents

Foreword | *Nina Teicholz*

Few people realize: A global revolution in nutrition is underway. For more than half a century, the populations of many nations have followed basic dietary recommendations to avoid fat and cholesterol as the best measure of prevention against disease. This advice, first launched by the American Heart Association in 1961 and enshrined as fact by the US Dietary Guidelines in 1980, is finally coming to an end. At the same time, scientists and researchers have gained a new perspective in understanding nutrition-related diseases. People everywhere are discovering that the surest way to improve health and reverse disease is, paradoxically, by ignoring the guidelines.

To put this in food terms, fat is no longer the enemy. Instead, according to a sizable body of rigorous scientific evidence, a diet somewhat higher in fat and lower in carbohydrates than the currently recommended norm turns out to be more effective for obtaining and maintaining good health.

The history of how we came to think that dietary cholesterol and fat are bad for health is an almost unbelievable story. In the late 1950s, a small group of US scientists, noting a correlation between blood plasma lipoproteins and heart disease, extrapolated that dietary fat must be to blame. They proposed the idea that a "heart healthy" diet meant shunning natural fats and cholesterol-rich foods, such as butter and red meat, in favor of industrially produced margarine and vegetable oils instead. Some of these researchers worked closely with the vegetable oil industry, which no doubt influenced their thinking, but they were also true believers in their so-called "diet-heart" hypothesis. The idea that saturated fats and cholesterol were unhealthy answered an urgent question at the time—what *did* cause this new and fast-rising condition called heart disease? The diet-heart hypothesis won the day.

Yet it is an astonishing fact that this hypothesis could never be shown to be true. Despite billions of dollars spent by governments around the world on randomized, controlled clinical trials—the "gold standard" of evidence—experiments on large populations could never demonstrate that fat *of any kind* had any effect on cardiovascular mortality, total mortality, or indeed any kind of nutrition-related

disease. In fact, the studies have not only revealed that the low-fat diet is ineffective at fighting chronic disease, but that in some cases it actually *worsened* a number of heart-disease risk factors. In other words, the low-fat diet actually appears to cause some of the very conditions it was meant to prevent.

The story of how these findings came to be ignored or suppressed is, as the *Lancet* recently described it, one of "scientific incompetence, evangelical ambition, and ruthless silencing of dissent that has shaped our lives for decades."

Responding, finally, to the science, both the US government and the American Heart Association in recent years have backed out of their "low-fat" diet recommendations. Search their websites for "low-fat diet," and you come up with nothing current.

The failure of this strategy has spurred researchers to look elsewhere in the diet for causes of nutrition-related disease, and most of the promising new research focuses on the dangers of carbohydrates.

This new evidence, which basically turns the food pyramid on its head, is simply unbelievable to many. Yet for those suffering from obesity or type 2 diabetes, it can be a glimmer of hope in an otherwise bleak landscape promising nothing more than futile diets and progressively worsening diseases, often accompanied by an ever-increasing load of medications. A nutritional regime that is lower in carbohydrates, as described in the pages of this book, is one based on whole, natural foods and fats, without hunger or calorie counting. It is nothing less than a new paradigm in thinking about how to eat.

The authors of this book are the leaders of this new thinking in New Zealand. Their beautiful book is a unique combination of solid science, sumptuous recipes developed by a top chef, and a surfeit of practical, easy-to-read tips on how to implement a "low-carb, healthy fat" diet for improved well-being. For those embarking on the journey to better health, it is a smart, comprehensive companion.

Nina Teicholz – Science journalist and author of international and *New York Times* best seller *The Big Fat Surprise*

Introduction | *Pete Evans*

Congratulations! By taking the time to pick up *What the Fat?*, you've just opened up a whole new world: one in which you will take back your health and experience a total mind and body overhaul that will completely transform you. I say this with a lot of confidence because for me, minimizing my carbohydrate intake and increasing the amount of good-quality fats I eat has been an absolute game-changer. Now in my early forties, I'm fitter, faster, and stronger than I've ever been. *What the Fat?* is a book that lets you investigate the science behind this way of life and gives you a real understanding of why this lifestyle works so well – as well as conveying lots of practical tips and ideas so you can choose to eat this way each and every day.

Once I discovered that the food I choose to eat has an all-encompassing impact on the state of both my physical and my emotional health, there was no turning back. I can proudly say I'm in better shape than I've ever been before. I know this because I love to surf and I used to get tired after a couple of hours in the water, but now I can charge for six to seven hours without feeling fatigued. I'm also mentally sharper and have broken down massive personal barriers, all through eating nutrient-dense whole foods. Now I'm inspired to spread the message and help others all over the globe discover for themselves the power of food as medicine.

My own journey began thanks to my wife, Nic, who grew up on a farm just outside of Christchurch, New Zealand. Being raised as a rural Kiwi girl means that she's always been well connected to her food sources. There is an overwhelming body of nutritional research that confirms that eating lots of good-quality fats and minimizing damaging carbohydrates and refined sugars is the only way we can take back control of our health and the health of our planet. Taking this pathway also means you'll lose weight, get fit, and feel fantastic along the way. At its heart, *What the Fat?* is about encouraging us all to return to using local, seasonal ingredients, to eat nutrient-dense whole foods, and to live in a more sustainable and holistic way. And isn't this what we all want to achieve? To understand how to make the best possible choices for ourselves and our families?

If you are reading this book, I'm excited that you too are making the commitment to discovering the joy that comes from living a life of optimal health and well-being. Within these pages, Professor Grant Schofield, Dr. Caryn Zinn, and chef Craig Rodger have pulled together a whole lot of clear, concise, and practical information that will give you the nutritional roadmap you need to start your own journey. Because this is all about what's right for *you*.

That's why *What the Fat?* is such an important read when you are first starting out on your journey. By helping you understand the science behind the Low-Carb, *Healthy*-Fat (LCHF) approach and providing the practical tips needed to live this way each and every day, this book completely demystifies everything and will change the way you think.

Pete Evans – Award-winning chef, restauranteur, health coach, television presenter, and author

A new beginning

Heard the one about the fat professor, the whole-food dietitian, and the Michelin-trained chef who want to change the world?

Nope, this is not a silly joke. Far from it. In fact, we hope this book provides some serious answers. We hope it is the beginning of a life-changing journey for many who have experienced inexplicable weight gain, the heartbreak of constant deprivation and yo-yo dieting, or, worse, physical illness through poor nutrition. We believe it's time to change the game, and it starts right here with your willingness to turn the page and consider the science of the Low-Carb, *Healthy*-Fat (LCHF) lifestyle.

For decades, the brightest minds in the nutrition and science field have had fat pegged as the bad guy. As a result, many of us have been enslaved by an outdated food pyramid that has pushed us to eat carb-laden and processed food. As the evidence mounts against sugar and processed carbohydrates, it's time to flip the pyramid and break free of the fat phobia.

Our eyes have been opened to better science and better success stories in practice, with improved health outcomes for those who have previously struggled. It may seem extraordinary, but doing pretty much the exact opposite of the past fifty years of nutritional advice might be the answer to improved health for many. Going from high-carb, low-fat to Low-Carb, *Healthy*-Fat (LCHF) has helped us, our families, our friends, and our clients in a multitude of ways.

In this practical guide, we present inspiring success stories, compelling evidence, and simple ways to "eat upside-down." Forget everything you were taught at school, flip the food pyramid on its head, and start nourishing your body the way it was designed to be nourished.

Due to the science, we were willing to change our minds, and we now invite you to change yours. You have to be willing to think outside the square (or the pyramid, for that matter) to find what works for you, regardless of what the majority thinks.

Our mission in writing this book is to help you. We want to change the world. Join us in flipping the food pyramid and eating real food.

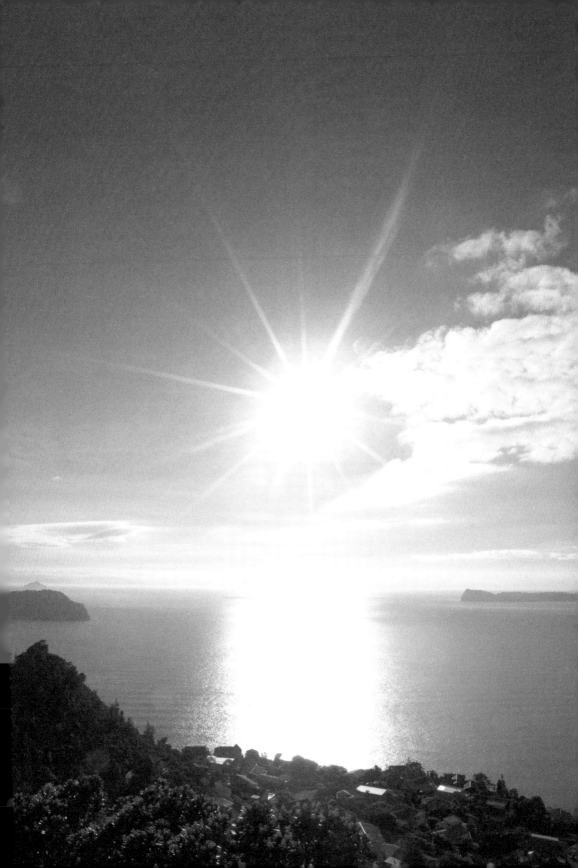

How to read this book

First up, if you are desperate to take your first step now, skip ahead to "The Skinny on LCHF" (page 14) – it's a short but not-so-sweet guide to what you can do right this minute. Then, take a deep breath, come back and read from here at your leisure.

We acknowledge that individuals come with a unique set of circumstances. This book is not intended to be a personalized diet plan, but rather an eating and lifestyle guide (including some science and lots of practice) as to how you and your family can embrace the LCHF lifestyle. For good. More importantly, the material provided in this book is not a substitute for medical care. We strongly recommend that you continue to seek appropriate advice from your physician, particularly if you're on medication.

The process of making a permanent change to the way you eat can take many months. This means you may need to return to *What the Fat?* several times. In fact, we encourage it. The book is constructed in such a way that you can read it in any order, so come back to any part of it as you please. Our advice to start with is to focus on the big-picture overview we present at the beginning ("The Skinny on LCHF," page 14), and then get started on making changes. Once you are underway, and noticing the results, you'll have lots of questions and will want to understand more about the science, and you'll appreciate the importance of topics that perhaps didn't make sense or weren't relevant the first time through.

In our experience, when you begin on the LCHF journey many of your friends and family will say things like "You're nuts" and "You have to be kidding" (a.k.a., "What the . . . ?") or "This is just the latest fad." But after a few weeks, when you are still going strong, they will begin to ask you lots (and lots) of questions – just give them a copy of this book. Once they start seeing your results, they will secretly start following LCHF. They will deny they ever questioned you.

During the course of this book we sometimes cover the same topic from different angles. This is because all three of us (like you) have our own unique story of how we came to understand and live the LCHF way of life. So there are three voices in *What the Fat?* In Part 1, the pronoun "I" refers to Caryn, our whole-food dietitian; in Part 2, "I" indicates that Craig, our Michelin-trained chef, is speaking; and, finally, in Part 3, "I" refers to Grant, our "Fat Professor." The pronoun "we" refers to all three of us (Caryn, Craig, and Grant) and represents our collective opinion or advice.

Now follow us on your journey into optimal well-being.

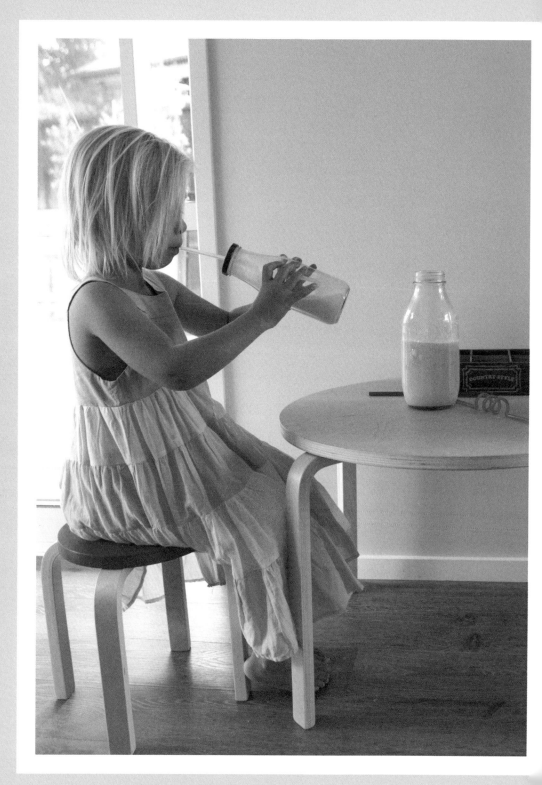

Life begins at 60

HELEN WOOD, 60

I turned sixty last July and was about to become a grandmother for the first time. I decided to tidy up my life, get healthy, and acquire some new information. I enrolled for a Level 1 + 2 First Aid Certificate course (covering cardio and infant) and started researching to find a diet that might actually work for me. I had long suspected that wheat and grain did not agree with my body and knew (with a handful of Smarties regularly inserted into my mouth) that I was totally hooked on sugar. After reading and reading . . . and reading some more, I came to the conclusion that the authors of *Cereal Killers*, *Wheat Belly*, and so many other books were onto something. So I embraced LCHF with gusto.

All osteoarthritis pain disappeared within a couple of weeks – I'm talking white-hot bolts through each knuckle, both ankles and feet, and my spine. All reflux and bloating disappeared within the same time frame. From sleeping propped up almost vertical on three or four pillows, numerous cushions, and neck rolls, for around five or six years, I can now happily sleep on one pillow like a normal person. All asthma has "left the building" – I no longer suck on puffers twice a day . . . and no more hairy tongue!

My brain is clear, sharp, and back to working as it used to, especially after giving up the statins that had been prescribed and were worse than useless, causing incredible muscle and tissue pain.

And I shed 45 pounds of visceral fat – with great ease! I'm still researching and enjoying what I'm learning, and know I'll never, ever, ever be tempted to give up my LCHF lifestyle – I don't have a death wish!

Grandchildren are the best part of growing older.

The skinny on LCHF

This (skinny) section is the cheat's guide for those who wanted to start yesterday, or those who don't have time to read the whole book (at least right now – we suspect you'll be back!). Or even those who just want to know what all the fuss is about. Here we give you all the basics to help you get started, straight away.

What is LCHF?

- LCHF typically stands for Low-Carb, High-Fat, but we have renamed it Low-Carb, *Healthy*-Fat. We feel that this better reflects what it's all about. While we do want you to eat more fat than you are probably used to, the emphasis is on healthy sources of fat. LCHF is not a "diet"; it is a way of life. This book teaches you what you need to know to live the LCHF lifestyle; it covers the benefits you'll reap and the reasons behind the stunning successes from eating and living the Low-Carb, *Healthy*-Fat way. Come, join us!
- The LCHF lifestyle encompasses a way of eating that embraces whole foods – foods that are minimally processed and generally don't come in packages. If you truly embrace this way of eating, it will naturally end up being lower in carbohydrate and higher in fat than the current, mainstream way of eating. LCHF is a fulfilling and satisfying way of eating that is full of benefits for health. While there is an element of restriction (as there is with whatever you do in life), it is not about deprivation.

Why should YOU do it?

LCHF has many different advantages, both for yourself and for your family. Here are the top five you might identify with. Do you want to:

- Lose weight and keep it off for good? Have you tried to lose weight before and for a moment believed you were successful, but then put the weight back on again (along with some more)?
- Have a healthy relationship with food? Do you constantly feel hungry and beat yourself up when you eat foods you "shouldn't"?
- Improve inflammatory health conditions? Do you suffer from aches and pains and inflammation for which you have to rely on medications for improvements?
- Break free of that "tired and run-down" feeling? Do you have a busy lifestyle, feel permanently exhausted, and regularly end up reaching for quick, unhealthy food?
- Live better for longer? Do you simply want to "be the best you can be" in health and in life? Do you want to be able to provide food for yourself and your family that is tasty, nourishing, and easy?

If you find yourself nodding your head when you read this list, then LCHF is definitely for you.

Why LCHF works

- If you gain weight easily, feel lethargic and stressed, and are out of shape, chances are you are insulin resistant and intolerant to carbs (more detail about this later). LCHF is the best lifestyle approach for managing insulin resistance.
- When you can control your blood sugars and the hormones that control your energy levels and weight (especially insulin), your body will respond by working as it was designed to – as a fat-burning machine!
- Weight control will become effortless, your energy levels will be better and you will feel great – free at last from the low-fat calorie-counting way of living that left you hungry, sick, and tired.
- What raises glucose and insulin levels? Carbo-hydrate, of course. We all vary in how we respond to and tolerate carbs. Finding your particular carb-tolerance level means your blood sugar and insulin will be well controlled.

What will I eat?

- Good-quality carbs from whole foods that are minimally processed, such as vegetables (lots of non-starchy ones), fruit, dairy products, and the occasional legume (beans and peas).
- Protein from minimally processed meat, fish, chicken, eggs, dairy products, nuts, seeds, and legumes.
- Fat from whole, minimally processed plant and animal sources, including avocado, olive oil, nuts, fatty fish, dairy products, and coconut products.

What shouldn't I eat?

- Refined and processed junk foods containing sugar.
- Refined, nutrient-poor, packaged carbohydrate-based foods, including most grains, such as breads, cereals, pasta, rice, granola bars, and crackers.

The 10 rules

01 Go low "HI"
Replace processed foods with stuff that was recently alive - foods low in the Human Interference (HI) factor. Real, actual food is the foundation of the LCHF lifestyle.

02 Cut the carbs (down . . . not out)
Sugar and grains are not good for you (yes, that means bread, even if it is wholegrain). Just how low you go depends on your personal tolerance to carbs, or degree of insulin resistance.

03 Virtuous vegetables
Vegetables are good for you. Eat lots of them, at each meal if possible. The good news is you can add fats such as olive oil or butter to make them taste even better.

04 Make fat your friend
Sugar is out, total carbs are low, protein is moderate, and, because you have to get your energy from somewhere, fat is in. We will show you how to overcome "fat phobia."

05 Put protein in its place
You need protein for life - but once you have more than your body needs, it gets converted into sugars by the liver. LCHF is not a high-protein diet. Many people stall in their progress because they are overdoing the protein.

06 Eat on cue
The whole point of LCHF is that your body will now be able to send and receive the messages it needs to stay in shape, to tell you when you are full, and to energize you.

07 Sort your support
Other people matter. Surround yourself with helpers, ask for support, and don't be afraid to request exactly what you want when you are out and about. Yes, it feels odd to order a burger without the bun the first time, but you will be amazed at how much people will help someone on a life mission.

08 Diligence, not effort
Relying on your "won't power" (effort) - like avoiding the chocolate cookies in your pantry - is futile. Instead, rely on being organized and having a ready supply of the right foods around you (diligence) in the first place.

09 Adopt the "three-meal" rule
You, like us, are human. Humans make mistakes. We do, and we expect you will fall off the wagon. That's okay, as long as we can help you jump back on again. We run the three-meal rule: there are three meals a day, 21 meals in a week. Let's get most of them right, knowing that three meals off the wagon a week is okay.

10 It's not just about the food
News flash from the Professor and Doctor Obvious: other things also affect your health - exercise, booze and cigarettes, drugs, stress, sleep, and much more. We will help you understand how these fit (or don't fit) into the LCHF lifestyle.

Our top-three FAQs

Will LCHF be bad for my health?

No, the exact opposite. Eating nutrient-dense whole foods with good-quality fats, while reducing nutrient-poor carbohydrate foods, promotes good health and may even reduce or eliminate some existing health issues.

Is LCHF a fad diet?

Definitely not. LCHF more closely mimics what humans have been eating the entire time they have been on the planet. It helps work around some of the problems of modern life that cause insulin resistance and then poor health. The real "problem diet" is the one recommended by the current nutritional guidelines promoting a low-fat, high-carb way of eating that causes more harm than good. Just look at the world's obesity and diabetes stats.

How can a diet that eliminates an entire nutrient be legitimate?

Firstly, we don't eliminate an entire nutrient. Fat and protein are essential nutrients, meaning the body cannot produce them – without them, we get sick and die. However, carbohydrate is not an essential nutrient and the body produces enough for our needs. So we encourage a reduction in carbs from the massive amount modern humans eat. We definitely include some carb foods, such as fruit, vegetables, and dairy products. These foods also provide a rich source of other great nutrients, such as fiber, vitamins, and minerals, and are good sources of good-quality protein and fat. Foods such as pasta, rice, crackers, breads, and cereals provide little nutrient value, i.e., very few micronutrients (vitamins and minerals), and minimal protein and fat. These are clearly not the best sources of carbs for the body.

Just one day eating the LCHF way

Here's a snapshot of a typical day eating the LCHF way.

BREAKFAST	LUNCH	DINNER	SNACK
Omelette with bell pepper, tomato, mushrooms, spinach, and cheese (cooked in olive oil, butter, or coconut oil)	*Salad* with a range of veggies, including leafy greens, canned salmon, avocado, nuts, and seeds and an olive oil–based dressing	*Steak* with blue-cheese sauce served on zucchini "noodles," green beans, and carrots drizzled with olive oil	*Berries* with yogurt and/or cream

Like anything done well in life, the devil is in the details – that's why we have combined not only the what (to do), but more importantly the how (you can achieve it), and finally the why (you would do it). This book is designed to be the definitive tell-me-everything-I-need-to-know guide to living the LCHF lifestyle.

Diabetes averted: 37-pound weight loss without effort

GARY BRIDGER, 63, AIR NEW ZEALAND A320 CAPTAIN

The triggers that led me to LCHF were a steady increase in weight and a rising blood-sugar count whenever I had my Commercial Pilot Licence medical check. Pilots are generally very health-conscious; our continued employment depends on it. If you end up with diabetes, that's the end of being a pilot. Fellow pilot and long-term friend Gary Hayman convinced me of the perils of excessive sugar in our diet, so I started off by drastically cutting down on sugar. The results were a 13-pound drop in weight, but little change to the rising blood-sugar levels. I was perilously close to Type 2 diabetes, and to being unemployed.

It was only then that I visited Dr. Caryn Zinn, who put me on a carb-restricted, healthy-fat diet to lower my blood sugar levels and further reduce my weight. She also got me to download an app for my iPhone for tracking my carb and protein intake (Easy Diet Diary). Following Caryn's eating plan, the results were immediate and dramatic. After three months eating the low-carb way, I had lost another 24 pounds (37 pounds total) and my HbA1c blood-sugar reading had gone from "prediabetic" to "normal."

I have been absolutely delighted with the results and am committed to LCHF eating long term. Fortunately, I have had excellent support from my wife and family, who have also embraced the new way of eating. This whole experience has been a huge benefit to me. Just having my weight and blood-sugar levels under control not only gives me the security of employment, but also makes me feel much more energetic than before. Because I have benefited so much, I have continued to spread the word among fellow pilots, family, and friends. Many have taken up the challenge and all have had similar results.

The hardest part of LCHF eating for me was finding suitable meals at work and away from home. Many cafés simply don't offer LCHF options, but with a little imagination you can adapt. For example, a Caesar salad without the croutons is a good solution, or a burger and salad and just leave the bun and fries. I also take small packets of nuts with me as snacks to tide me over until I can find suitable meal options.

For favorite foods, I do enjoy breakfast with eggs, bacon or sausage, mushrooms, and green vegetables for a good start to the day. That breakfast for me is the key, and keeps me going nicely until lunchtime. For lunch, always a salad at home. Family evening-meal favorites include roast lamb and ratatouille with cauliflower mashed with butter, thickened cream, and Parmesan cheese. Other favorites are lasagne with sliced zucchini instead of pasta and "potato top" pie with mashed cauliflower instead of potato. We have been eating more fish than before and, of course, more "above ground" vegetables. I have also been cooking Malaysian (our favorite ethnic food) chicken or fish curries with plenty of added vegetables and cauliflower rice instead of conventional rice – divine!

12 key terms you need to understand

In *What the Fat?* we will use some terms you might have heard of, and others you may not have. Here we list the 12 key terms essential to getting the most out of this book.

01 **Insulin** is part of a complex hormonal and neural system that affects all parts of our body. Insulin is a protein hormone produced by the pancreas. It helps in the regulation of nutrients and energy around the body. It is best known for helping move glucose (carbs) into cells so that it can be used for energy. That's a crucial function – without insulin you will die. Type 1 diabetes is a failure of the pancreas to produce insulin. To survive, Type 1 diabetics must inject synthetic insulin.

02 If you are **insulin sensitive**, then insulin works in low amounts to move glucose into your cells for energy.

03 If you are **insulin resistant**, then it is hard for insulin to open your cells to receive glucose. So your body will need lots of insulin to achieve the same thing as an insulin-sensitive person.

04 **Metabolically dysregulated** is a term used to describe someone who is insulin resistant as a result of their poor lifestyle. The body is out of its normal operative mode and stores energy as fat easily, and does not easily burn fat.

05 **Fat adapted** or "metabolically flexible" are terms we use to describe people who can easily burn fat as a primary fuel source, and use the by-products (ketones) as an energy source when carbs are low in their diet.

06 **Ketones** are an important fuel source for humans when glucose (carb) supply is low. Ketones can be used by the brain, organs, and muscle. When you become fat adapted (or metabolically flexible), it really means that your body is learning how to use ketones as a fuel. People with high-carb diets hardly ever have to use this system, so the body requires some re-orchestration when going through this process.

07 **Carbohydrates** (carbs) are found in many foods, but exist in high levels in starchy and sugary foods and refined and processed modern foods. This includes breads and cereals, pasta, potatoes, rice, sugar, and honey. Carbohydrates mostly break down into glucose, the simplest carbohydrate in the body. Although we need glucose to live, the body can produce enough of its own through various means, so eating carbs is not essential for life.

08 **Protein** (made up of amino acids) is essential for life, and we have to get many of the "essential" amino acids from food because the body cannot produce them.

09 **Fat** is a component of the whole foods we see as being part of a healthy diet. Fat comes in different types and sub-types. Most of us have heard of the basic types: monounsaturated, polyunsaturated, and saturated.

10 **Monounsaturated fats** are high in foods such as olive oil.

11 **Polyunsaturated fats** are high in some plant foods, such as nuts and seeds, and all sorts of animal foods, including fish. There are two types of polyunsaturated fat that are called "essential fatty acids" – omega-3 and omega-6. These cannot be produced by the body and must be obtained through eating foods containing them.

12 **Saturated fats** are higher in animal foods, such as meats and dairy, but are also in some plant-based foods, such as coconut oil. Most foods as they occur in nature have a combination of all fats. For example, lard is about one-third each monounsaturated, polyunsaturated, and saturated fat.

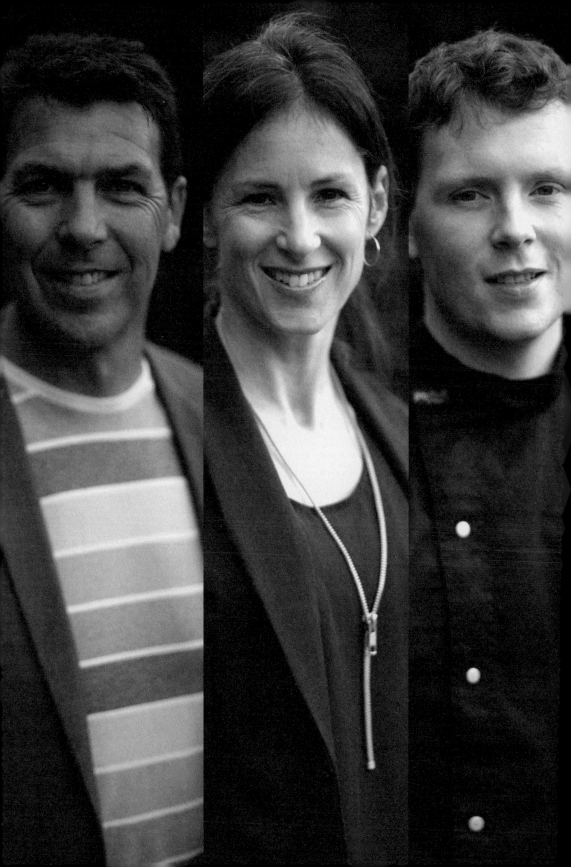

Our stories

We are all different. We understand that every individual comes with their own personal story and that is part of who they are. In this section, we invite you to read our stories and hope that you connect with our mission and our philosophies about food.

The "Fat Professor"

PROFESSOR GRANT SCHOFIELD

I have become known as the "Fat Professor." I'm not fat, although I can easily put weight on, especially whenever I stop serious exercise. I'm the Fat Professor because I have been strongly advocating a major rethink about the way we view our food, and especially fat, in our society. I believe that the modern dietary guidelines, the modern food supply, and the way in which a great deal of nutrition science is conducted needs a serious rethink. We need a new focus on nourishing, sustainable, and satisfying food. We need a relationship with food that helps us be the best version of ourselves. Part of that will be letting go of the low-fat mantra and embracing fat in the context of food from whole plants and animals. That's right, I'm advocating that we eat more fat! My entire research and practice career has centered around understanding what helps us be the best we can be. That's what has inspired the broad description of my research, practice, and blog, "The Science of Human Potential." Besides my team's work in challenging nutritional conventions, we have also become well known for our work in rethinking modern (sitting) work environments, using standing desks to give both health and productivity benefits. Moving more at work provides a classic win–win situation for employers and employees. I've coined the term GOYA to describe it – getting off your arse and moving more!

Our work in rethinking children's play has also generated an unprecedented amount of media and public comment. Like our work in diet and health, it's not so much about an original idea, but about having the guts to point out the obvious. The obvious here is that kids no longer take risks and play in the outdoors in the way they used to. The "free-range

kid" is an endangered species. Our work has shown the benefits, and now the public appetite, for children to have the sort of childhood that is normal – one where risk, play, and adventure are experienced on their own terms without adults. I'm describing a childhood where they can run amok and make their own mistakes. Doesn't it make total sense that to develop brains that can cope with stress, emotion, and risk, those same brains need exposure to stress, emotion, and risk? The great paradox of society's efforts to cocoon our children is that by protecting them we actually make them less safe in the long run. I'd say the appropriate time to experience risk is up a tree when you are eight years old, not when you are eighteen and driving a Subaru with your buddies egging you on and the police chasing you.

I've always tried to call things as they really are, not as convention wants to see them. I haven't always been that interested in food, though. In fact, many who knew me in my earlier days will tell you that I often described nutrition as being way less important for health than exercise. That was my research career – millions of dollars in competitive research grants, over 100 peer-reviewed publications, and being one of the youngest professors in New Zealand academia. My career was flying along; all I had to do was play the game and stick to exercise. Then, three good reasons rocked that status quo, prompting a complete change of heart.

Reason 1: Professional triathlete

I spent my younger years competing as a serious (professional) triathlete. Despite training up to thirty hours a week, maintaining a lean body weight was always a struggle for me. I followed the "healthy"

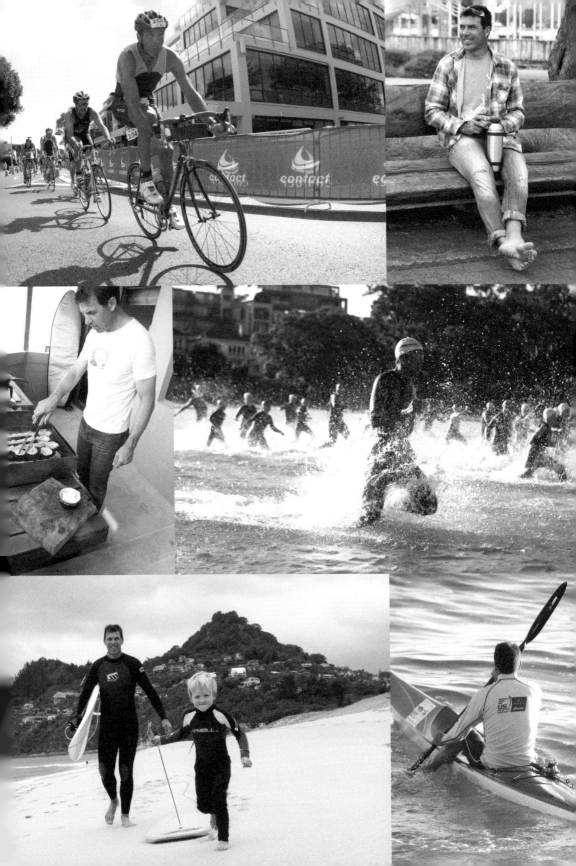

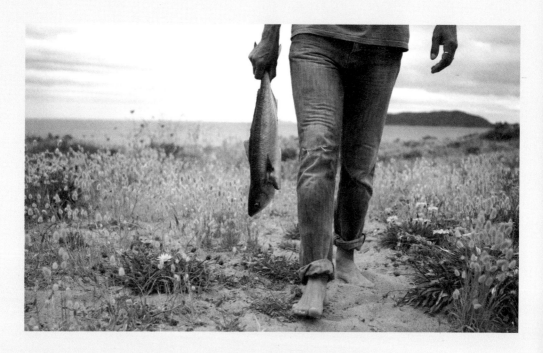

eating advice diligently: low on fat with all the carbs I needed to sustain my enormous energy output. I worked and trained wisely. I was very dedicated. Yet despite my discipline, my racing weight of 85-87 kg was just too heavy to compete at the highest level. Whenever I stopped that level of intense training, my weight tracked up fast. Very fast. After the birth of our second child, Jackson, in 2003, I reached 103 kg. I wasn't training nearly as much. Exercising once a day and eating healthily just wasn't enough to stop the insidious weight gain. It was obvious to me then that exercise was way more important than nutrition because exercise, excessive exercise, was the only thing that worked for me. Clearly something is not right about this picture – for me and for everyone else who must exercise excessively to keep their weight in check.

Reason 2: Futile research

I had run dozens of studies (including large randomized controlled trials in high-risk populations) aimed at reducing weight and improving cardio-metabolic health, yet nothing really worked. In public health, we spend millions telling people to eat less, reduce fat, and move more. But it is clear to me now that something is wrong with that message. Most people assume that weight gain and poor health are due to failing to stick to the guidelines, not that it's the guidelines and science itself that is wrong.

Reason 3: Working in the Pacific Islands

When I was under contract to the World Health Organization across the South Pacific islands, working to prevent diabetes and noncommunicable diseases, it became obvious that the people who ate the most fat were often the healthiest. The people relying on processed carbs were in the worst shape. Walking around spouting the World Health Organization recommendations, telling people to "eat less and move more," suddenly struck me as ridiculous. Putting all the responsibility and blame on the individual's willpower (or lack thereof) just misses the underlying biology of the problem. The problem in the Pacific is refined and processed carbohydrates, which Pacific people are not designed to eat in any quantity. Reading nutritional anthropology of traditional societies (Weston A. Price's accounts of dental health and Vilhjalmur Steffanson's *My Life with the Eskimo*) made me realize that what has worked for humans the entire time they've been on the planet has absolutely nothing to do with the so-called "healthy" food pyramid.

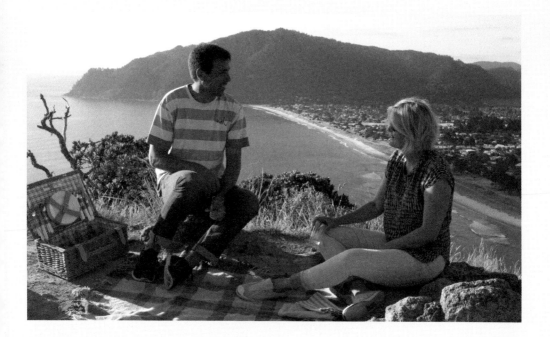

To sum up

We have a lot to learn from our ancestors. Our wish to discard traditional knowledge and practices in the name of science is fundamentally flawed. Sure, science can answer questions. But science is always just a set of hypotheses – and hypotheses can be proven wrong at any point. It's been said that half of what we know in science is wrong; we just need to figure out which half. I think that's especially true of nutrition science, a science still in its infancy.

I am now convinced that mainstream nutrition science and practice is based more on dogma, industry-vested interest, academics "playing the game" to get their research grants and publications, and people playing it safe for a safe career. I know how to play those games; I have played those games. Well, now I'm taking my ball and I'm not playing with those kids anymore. We are changing the rules. In a brave new world, where ivory-tower academics are less relevant and everyone has access to information through the Internet, the rise of the intelligent blogger with no vested interest has led us into a new nutrition dimension. Thankfully, the rules and the field have changed forever.

As a scientist, I believe that it's my job to be curious, to investigate other possibilities, and to be willing to change my mind. I have to pursue the truth regardless of what the majority thinks. That's been the biggest challenge, and it still is. Wherever I go, people say to me, "Virtually every eminent scientist in the world thinks fat, especially saturated fat, is bad for you, Professor Schofield. Who are you to say otherwise?" But science isn't a popularity contest; it isn't a democracy. Like Nobel laureate Richard Feynman, I believe that "science alone of all the subjects contains within itself the lesson of the danger of belief in the infallibility of the greatest teachers of the preceding generation." The preceding generation gave us a food pyramid prescribing a high-carb, low-fat diet. But my personal experience and professional research has convinced me that this prescription is wrong. By eating more like our ancestors, we can halt the obesity epidemic and reverse our own expanding waistlines.

The whole-food dietitian

DR. CARYN ZINN

My story as an L*CHF*, whole food-advocate dietitian has come about from being a reflective practitioner and a critical thinker, and from making an honest acknowledgment that we have simply got it wrong.

I have been in dietetic practice for around 20 years and have always considered myself fairly conservative in my approach as a dietitian. My day-to-day work involves teaching, research, and practice. Until two years ago, this work aligned with my country's national nutrition guidelines, which advocate a high-carbohydrate, low-fat way of eating. Because of our growing obesity epidemic, the supposed logic behind my "guideline loyalty" was to live by the energy-balance equation and limit nutrients that provided a lot of calories, i.e., fat.

During the past few years of my career, I have come to the conclusion that we have got it wrong. I have subsequently made a complete 180-degree change of direction in my nutritional philosophies, and my practice. This was not an easy thing to do. During this time, I was so confused about what was right and what was wrong, and angst-ridden as to what I should be teaching and practicing with my clients, that I even considered changing my profession. But extensive reading and critiquing, self-guinea-pigging, and cautious experimentation with some willing clients quashed my doubts. I had been using low carb in my approach with clients for years, but not high fat (particularly animal fat) – so the first time I instructed a client to buy full-fat cheese and milk, and to be liberal with their use of olive oil, my hair stood on end.

Here's why I changed my mind and why I've never looked back. I'd been wondering: Why has our approach over the past 50 years simply not worked? Why are we getting less healthy? Finally, I applied the three pieces of the puzzle – evidence, practice, and logic – and it all fell into place.

Reason 1: Evidence

I have been more open to reading research on low-carbohydrate, high-fat nutrition. I had disregarded this in the past (it went against the conventional wisdom!) – but now, with my eyes open, I find it is much more compelling than the flawed research that resulted in our national guidelines. Call it career maturity or just "timing," who knows? Could it be coincidental that since the carb-focused, low-fat nutrition guidelines were officially adopted in 1977, we have as a nation become fatter and sicker? More than one-third of adults and almost 20 percent (one-fifth) of children are obese on a global scale, with diabetes rife, and both obesity and diabetes rates are climbing.

The science of L*CHF* nutrition shows that this way of eating is a viable and healthy option for many people. Not only does it include more nutrient-dense whole-food sources, but it is also excellent for weight loss and can be useful in helping people with a range of serious medical conditions, from diabetes and cancer to Alzheimer's.

Reason 2: Practice

I have reflected on my clinic-based practice as a dietitian, particularly with my weight-loss clients. With the mainstream low-fat approach, clients do lose weight – but they do so with constant feelings of hunger and the need to incorporate immense amounts of exercise to keep the weight off, which is just not sustainable.

The problem with mainstream low-fat practice is that dietitians, who are by and large slim individuals, think that if the food we're eating works for us, then surely it should work for our clients. Unfortunately, this notion is totally wrong; the reality is that the same food can have profoundly different metabolic effects on different people, and, perversely, the people we

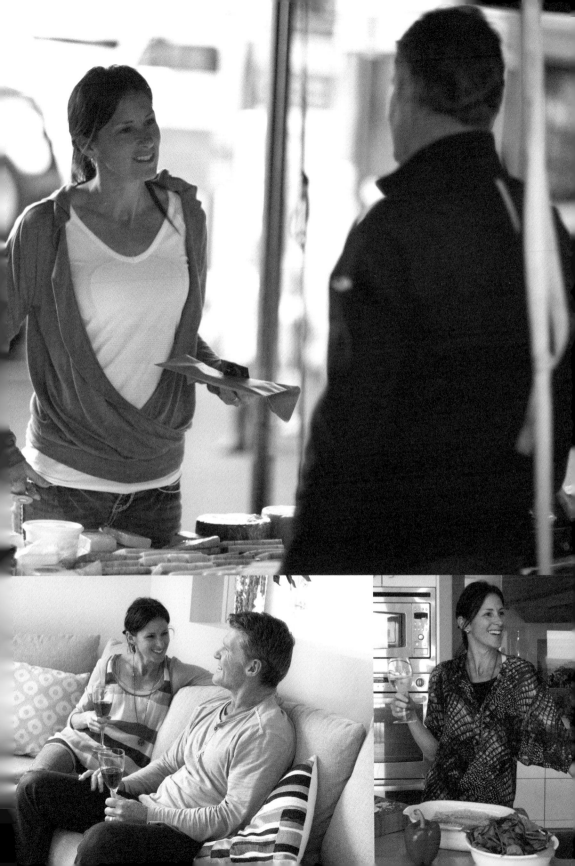

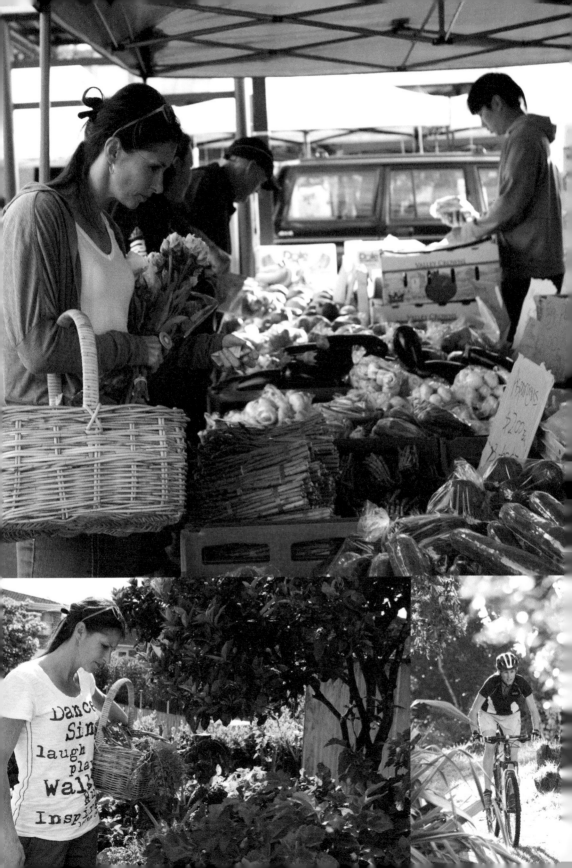

want to help the most benefit the least from the low-fat approach.

My practice using LCHF has resulted in an incredible (unprompted) array of success stories of increased energy, better sleep, improved moods, reduced gut issues, improved skin conditions, and reduced inflammatory conditions. All this while not feeling hungry, claiming that the LCHF way of life is easy, and exercising for general health rather than for the sole purpose of controlling weight. I've since seen friends, colleagues, and family all thrive eating in this whole-food, LCHF way.

Reason 3: Logic

It just doesn't seem logical to base our diet on foods that have been on this earth for a fraction of time compared with foods present since the beginning of time. Our ancient ancestors ate whole plant- and animal-based foods that contained little carbohydrate and sugar, and contained a lot of natural fat, and they suffered little chronic disease. Our packaged, processed, fortified food supply has done us harm and will continue to do harm if we don't take a stand and advocate for change. When so many of us experience conditions of insulin resistance (prediabetes, diabetes, polycystic ovary syndrome, and excess weight), it defies logic to manage these conditions with a diet high in the very nutrient that is at the center of the problem – i.e., carbohydrates.

To sum up

I have no "health story" to tell. I'm not overweight, never have been; I'm healthy and I am one of those fortunate people who can tolerate carbohydrate (well, at the moment anyway). So my reasons for change are purely about wanting to maintain "optimal" health – or being as healthy as I can possibly be. I love eating the LCHF way. For me, one of the greatest benefits is that I am just not hungry between meals, and this brings with it a huge feeling of calm – this is the best way I can describe it. I am now not scrambling for my next high-carb, 99 percent fat-free, packaged meal almost immediately after the last. This, along with knowing that I'm putting top-quality, nutrient-dense, delicious food into my body to fuel my cells, makes it easy to stick to. Even if weight loss is not your goal, even if you can tolerate a high-carbohydrate load now, this doesn't mean you have to, or that you will always be able to. It also doesn't mean that you couldn't do better with fewer carbs.

As I said at the start, my story as an LCHF, whole-food-advocate dietitian has come about from being a reflective practitioner, and a critical thinker, and from making an honest acknowledgment that we have simply got it wrong. Since my change in direction, I have been sharing my story with dietitians both in New Zealand and further afield. I have been presenting the LCHF science and outcomes from my practice to them in many different forums, and this has been met with a mixed response!

We, as dietitians, are a conservative group of health professionals in general, which is a good thing in some ways. For some, we need to be patient to allow such a drastic change in nutrition thinking and direction to sink in. In the meantime, I will continue to spread the word.

The Michelin-trained chef

CHEF CRAIG RODGER

Growing up on the west coast of Scotland, near Glasgow, I saw food as sustenance and fuel. The traditional Scottish food was potatoes, oat porridge, lentils, and barley soup. Stodge, we called it. It wasn't too inspiring, or nutritious for that matter. Watching the French master chefs demonstrate their art form on television was a fascinating departure from the food and the culture I grew up with. After a couple of unsuccessful ventures into tertiary education, I realized I wanted to get hands-on learning in the craft of cooking. I studied for three years at culinary college, where I learned the classical French repertoire of cooking. I embraced the food and the life of a chef, working at a four-star hotel for forty hours per week alongside my studies, and loved it. When college finished, I decided "finishing school" would be at a Michelin restaurant. I sent applications to the twelve restaurants in Scotland that had at least one Michelin star at the time, and I successfully interviewed for the first one that got back to me.

The reasons I ended up becoming an LCHF chef are simple, but they begin with a personal health scare.

Reason 1: Pre-diabetic at 28

I spent the next eighteen months working fourteen-hour days, six days a week – exactly what I had wanted at the time. I loved the standards and dedication to cooking and began to realize that the job of any chef, not least a chef aiming to excel, is to elicit pleasure in the diner, whatever the cost. I put this into practice when making a soufflé one day – you wouldn't want to know how much sugar was in the mix. I used the most stunningly sweet meringue-like egg mixture to produce a sweet-sour delight. Remember: elicit pleasure in the diner, whatever the cost. I figured that this was just the way things were and if I had any hope of achieving excellence in cooking, I just had to fall into line.

After moving to New Zealand with my Kiwi fiancée, I was inspired by those around me to get a thorough check-up from the doctor. I should have been more shocked at the diagnosis of "prediabetic" at the age of 28 – but after taste-testing hundreds of batches of soufflé (and myriad other sugary delights), I was far from surprised. At the age of 28, I was too young to just cave in to this reality. So I began to investigate whether I, as a chef, could cook and eat myself better.

Reason 2: My own research and reading

Apart from my medical diagnosis, my life in New Zealand was going well. My new family was very excited to have a chef in the mix. By this time, I'd been actively studying all the information available on the LCHF approach and had attended a seminar fronted by Professor Grant Schofield and Dr. Caryn Zinn. I read some books and implemented the approach to eating in my fiancée's life and mine. In the lead-up to our wedding, it was an invaluable tool for helping me regain my health (and my waistline) in time for our big day.

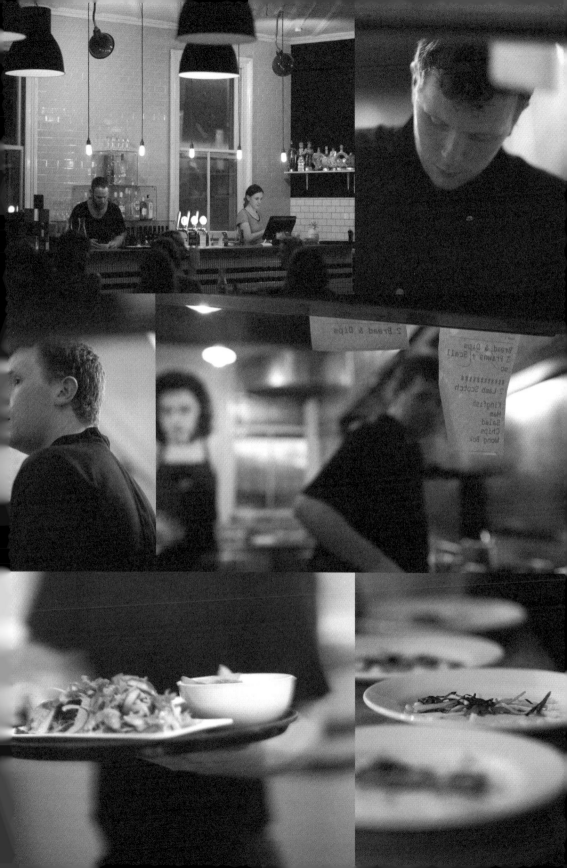

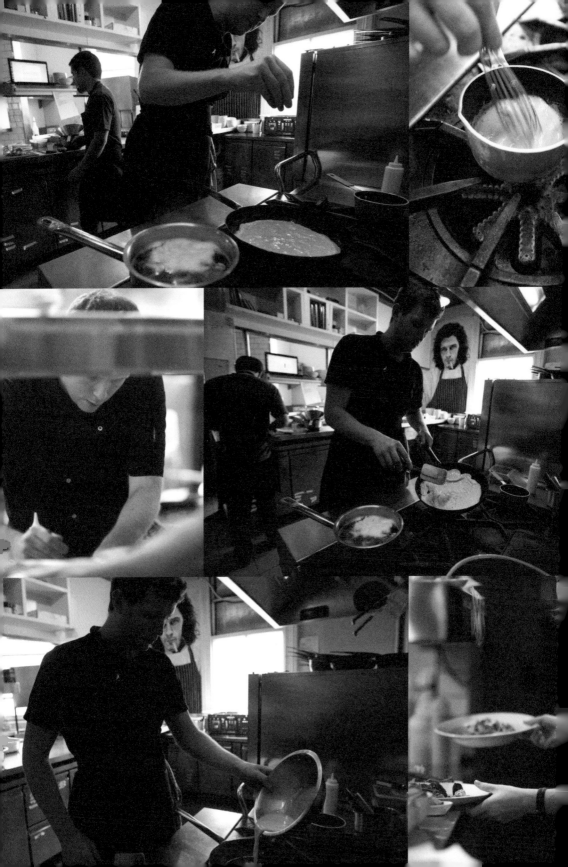

To sum up

The family was supportive of the slowly emerging idea that we, as a family, might open a restaurant one day. With my brother-in-law, Elliot, and my wife, Hailey, we had the makings of a team ready to take on the challenges of starting a restaurant with a twist. LOOP opened in April 2014, the result of an eight-month mission to find the right location for realizing our ideas. The restaurant was to feature seasonal and local food; the produce had to be ethically sourced and sustainable. Above all, the food had to be delicious and make people want to come back for more.

Naturally, down to my own experience, I wanted the cooking and recipes to rely on lower-carbohydrate options and to emphasize good nutrition. Some of the dishes I designed were entirely LCHF compliant, so that at least 25 percent of our first menu at LOOP featured strict LCHF options. The rest was built around whole foods, with an emphasis on nutrition and on staying away from unnecessary grains and filler foods as much as possible. I created a menu at LOOP to help spread the LCHF message – by offering top-quality, nutritious meals to our guests.

I've got my high-school weight back at 53!

CINDY WIERSMA, 53, SENIOR LECTURER

Eighteen months ago, I did the exact opposite of everything I have been told about nutrition. I flipped the food pyramid. My life has changed for good (really!) now that I am on LCHF. All the (healthy?) whole grains are out – butter, cream, and bacon are in.

The old

My diet usually consisted of cereal with skim milk for breakfast, a bread-based lunch, lots of pasta- and rice-based dinners, and a few too many snacks to get me through the day. I was snacking because I was hungry. Although I had no apparent health or weight issues, the few extra pounds sneaking on over the years meant that I had a growing number of clothes hanging in the closet that I no longer felt comfortable wearing. I also knew the difference between how people see you in clothes and how you look naked.

Time to change

I changed my HCLF (High-Carb, Low-Fat) diet to the LCHF real-food approach after seeing Grant and Caryn's initial LCHF seminar at the AUT Millennium high-performance sports facility. The evidence was compelling and it just made sense. I used a free diet app (Easy Diet Diary) for the first few months, which gave me a better understanding of what is in different foods, and have since used friends, books, and good old Google to find lots of simple, tasty LCHF recipes and ideas.

Now

My typical daily breakfast now consists of either eggs and veggies or unsweetened full-fat yogurt with berries and a scrumptious nuts/seeds mix for breakfast (it beats my old processed and expensive cereal hands down). I have an elaborate salad for lunch – lots of greens and veggies plus various combinations of egg, avocado, lightly toasted walnuts or pumpkin seeds, blue cheese, tuna/salmon/ham/chorizo/ground beef and an olive oil dressing. Dinner is meat- and veggie-based, but with so many scrumptious and easy LCHF recipes and ideas now available, the options are almost endless. A personal favorite is a very simple chicken laksa made with coconut cream, red curry paste, and lots of veggies. Snacks, although not usually required, might consist of nuts, cheese, or fruit, and a bit of delicious dark chocolate most days as my perennial weakness.

When asked what the hardest part has been, I have to say it isn't hard at all – I just love it. I thought I would never have the time to make breakfast or lunches for work, but have found that as long as there is a variety of good, healthy food in the fridge, it only takes

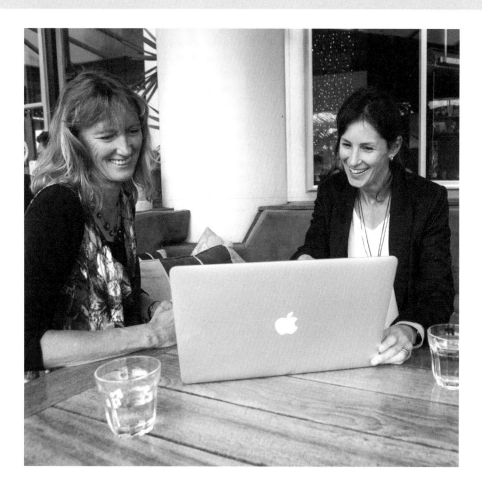

a minute to quickly grab bits and pieces, throw it into a plastic container and toss it together at work. After changing my diet, I probably missed bread and toast the most, but have since discovered some fantastic recipes for wheat-, grain-, and sugar-free breads which are super-easy and provide my fix of toast with butter or pesto and avocado. Yum!

I feel great, but then I never really felt unwell before either. However, one difference I have noticed is the absence of the late afternoon "weak and wobblies" – a term I used when I needed food badly towards the end of the day, especially if exercising. I often got to a point where I felt very weak all over and my legs would actually feel wobbly. I

used to explain it as "running out of calories" and I desperately needed a granola bar or chocolate bar at that stage. Although I can still feel hungry leading up to meal time, I no longer experience that sensation of crashing from lack of food as I did when carbohydrates were my main source of fuel.

I changed from HCLF to LCHF because I truly believed it was healthier and I was also hoping to shed a few pounds. I have never looked back. The pounds, 17 pounds, fell off without effort. The food is far nicer, I know it's healthier, and I feel great. I've had blood tests completed and everything is excellent. At 53, I feel fantastic, I love the food, and it's a real bonus to have my high-school butt back!

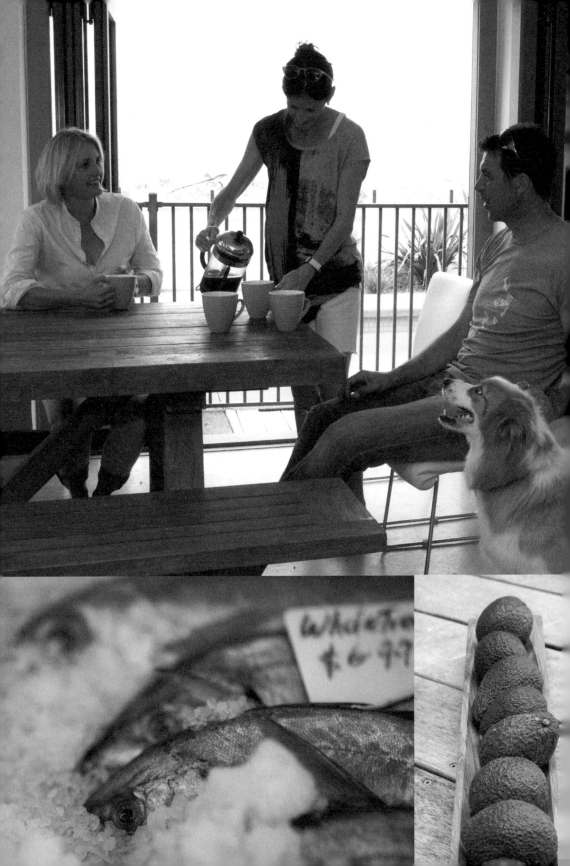

Part 1
Getting started with LCHF

Hi, it's me, Caryn.

In this section, I'm going to run you through the nuts and bolts of the LCHF lifestyle. We understand that embarking on a new way of eating prompts plenty of questions, so I plan to address these in a practical way 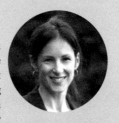 and provide you with all the advice you need to ensure that your meals are healthy and balanced, delivering optimal nutrition. That's my job!

The great thing for me about combining with Grant and Craig in *What the Fat?* is the diversity of knowledge we bring to the book. This is no ordinary cookbook where all you get is recipes and pretty pictures; in creating this book, we wanted to give you the whole picture on the LCHF lifestyle. Over the next pages I will walk you through the entire transition, covering how you are likely to feel, how you know whether LCHF is right for you, how to sort the pantry and set up the fridge, and, most important of all, how to make your new way of eating stick. No more diets, just natural and delicious whole food from here on in. No more calorie counting and, best of all, no more sweet tooth or constant hunger.

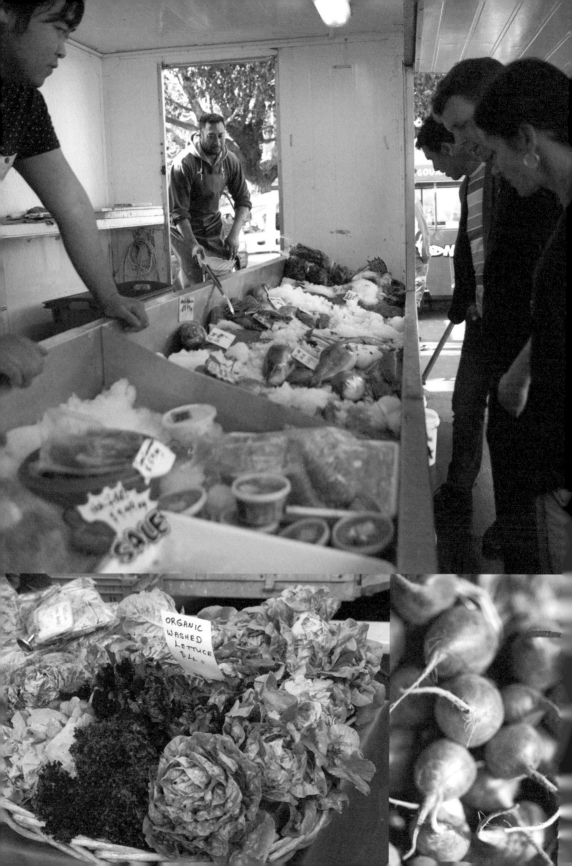

Is LCHF for me?

Have you ever wondered how much carbohydrate you eat on a daily basis?

Taking into consideration our modern food environment, where almost everything we eat is processed, packaged, and full of additives, and is laden with sugar and processed vegetable oils, we typically consume at least 250 g of carbohydrate each day. We have been encouraged (via our current national guidelines) to consume this amount, which is 45-65 percent of our total daily energy intake (i.e., the majority of our calories). Along with the "keep total fat intake low" guideline, the food industry has rubbed its hands together and manufactured a host of foods (or should I say items that resemble food) in convenient forms for us to meet these high-carb, low-fat guidelines. Shortly, I will tell you how to calculate how much carbohydrate (grams per day) you currently eat. You'll be surprised.

How much carbohydrate should I eat?

This is a fundamental question to consider when venturing into the LCHF lifestyle, and one you should spend a bit of time figuring out.

Firstly, since it's "low-carb," our basic premise is that you are going to adopt some level of carbohydrate restriction. I'll address how you go about reducing your carbohydrate load shortly, but first let's talk about how much carbohydrate might work for you.

There are various levels of carbohydrate restriction, and your personal level very much depends on your metabolic make-up, your goals, and your current circumstances. Unfortunately, I am unable to give you a personal prescription without knowing a whole lot more about you. However, I can tell you that carbohydrate restriction can largely be divided into two main categories: moderate restriction and extreme restriction.

Of course, if you currently have a very high intake of carbohydrate foods, you can simply eat less of them and you will still get a benefit. We usually find that once you start off doing this and become fascinated by the results, you'll want to consider the optimal levels of restriction for you as an individual. Ultimately, extreme carb restriction (ketogenic eating) is useful for a small proportion of the population, e.g., some athletes, individuals who are already eating LCHF but might have some lasting stubborn weight that needs to be lost, and potentially those with specific chronic illnesses, such as certain cancers and epilepsy.

Level of carbohydrate restriction	Amount of carbohydrate per day	Goal
Moderate restriction	Somewhere between 50 g and 100 g	Improved health, weight loss if needed
Extreme restriction ("ketogenic" eating)	Up to 50 g (initially 25-30 g)	Weight loss – stubborn body fat, treatment of conditions (cancer, epilepsy), endurance-sports performance

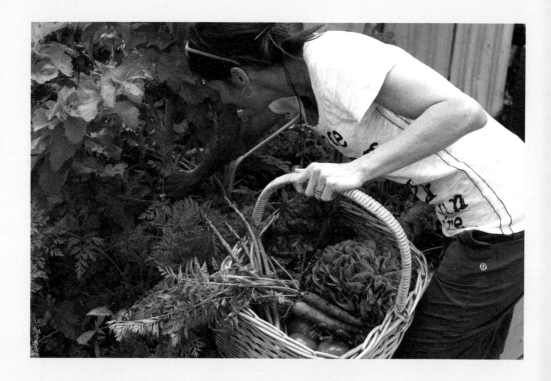

I believe that for many people, a moderate carbohydrate restriction is recommended; it is easy to do and is sustainable in the long term.

If you are intrigued as to what your current carb number is, you can accurately work this out using nutrition-analysis programs or apps on your smartphone or computer. I suggest you do this now, as you will learn a lot about where you find carbs in foods, as well as other macronutrients such as protein and fat. These programs are essential tools in a new LCHF lifestyle. They're invaluable for quickly checking the carb content of a food, or if you want to keep yourself on task, particularly at the start. There are many of these programs or apps around; some are better than others. Some incorporate food databases from New Zealand/Australia, and others include those from the US. Do be mindful with them, as one is not as accurate as the next. A good one for New Zealand and Australia is Easy Diet Diary, although unfortunately it is i-device only. FatSecret is another good one to use for all smartphones and computers, and is also available in South Africa. MyFitnessPal is a great one that is available in many countries.

Entering your daily food and fluid allows you to learn a great deal about macronutrients in food (i.e., carbs, protein, and fat) and what your daily totals amount to. Of course, if this activity seems a little onerous, you can just trust that if you typically eat according to the current guidelines (i.e., whole-grain breads and cereals, along with some other packaged foods), you are sure to be eating the average amount of carbohydrate (about 250 g or more).

Alternatively, find out if you need to restrict your carb intake (and to what level) by simply taking our carb-tolerance test (see opposite).

TAKE OUR TEST!

The carb-tolerance test

For each statement, give yourself a score between 1 and 5 and then add up the points.

1 = not true **2** = seldom true **3** = occasionally true **4** = mostly true **5** = definitely true

○ Dieting is hard for me because I get so hungry

○ I often feel so hungry that I have to eat something

○ I would describe myself as having a "sweet tooth"

○ I easily put on weight and it mostly goes on around my tummy (men) or hips (women)

○ I struggle to lose weight and keep it off

○ I am always hungry enough to eat any time

○ I always eat all the food on my plate, and often have seconds

○ When I'm hungry, I crave carbohydrate foods – especially sweet or starchy foods

○ I have close relatives with diabetes, gout, or heart disease

○ I would exercise more, but mostly feel sluggish and unmotivated

○ I am quite overweight, even though I have dieted a lot during my life

○ I have one or more of the following conditions: prediabetes, diabetes, gout, a neurological condition, arthritis or another inflammatory condition, gut-related disorders including celiac disease and IBS (by the way, if you score 5 [definitely true] on this statement alone, you will definitely benefit from the LCHF lifestyle).

Your score will be between 12 and 60

12-27

You are probably highly carbohydrate tolerant and can choose where to set your carbohydrate limit. Quitting sugar is a no-brainer, but the level of overall carbohydrate restriction is your choice from here.

28-43

You might have some carbohydrate intolerance, but it's not out of control just yet. You could benefit from some carbohydrate restriction by simply reducing your current level or going for moderate restriction.

44-60

You are almost certainly carbohydrate intolerant and stand to benefit from a moderate restriction of carbs using LCHF.

Surprised? We thought you might be . . . so hop on board and let's get started!

Getting fat adapted

Fat adaptation is what happens when your body shifts from being a carbohydrate fuel burner (which many of us are) to being a fat burner; i.e., it has adapted to using fat as a primary fuel source – ideally excess body fat, if you have it. Although the benefits of an LCHF lifestyle can often be seen in a matter of days, it is only once your body re-learns how to use fat as a fuel source, and you reach the point of fat adaptation, that you will start to experience the full set of beneficial outcomes. These can include effortless and stable energy levels, weight management (if that's the goal), and, for active individuals, the ability to perform and recover more efficiently and effectively. We call this "getting fat adapted."

The spectrum of fat adaptation is a little like the spectrum of carb restriction in that if you choose to restrict your carbs moderately, you will be moderately fat adapted, and if you choose to go whole hog and try the ketogenic diet, you will experience full fat adaptation.

Most people will experience the health and weight-control benefits they want and need with moderate fat adaptation or carb restriction, and for the majority of people this may be the best level. So I wouldn't recommend you go to the extreme of becoming fully fat adapted if you're achieving your goals in the middle of the spectrum. There is no point, and it might not be the right place for you anyway.

Whichever level you decide is suitable, there are several important nuances which can stop you from getting there, put you in a "feeling below par" metabolic grey zone as you get there, or cause other issues once you have got there. Here's what to look out for and how to avoid these traps.

Smooth sailing into carb restriction

Be prepared. It's likely that you will experience some (or all) of these symptoms if you have been on a moderate- to high-carb diet (anything over 250 g per day) and you switch over to an LCHF whole-food diet:

- Lack of energy
- Sweet cravings
- Light-headedness
- Constipation
- Dizziness
- Brain fog

These symptoms are temporary and some people don't experience them at all. The severity of your symptoms and the likelihood of getting them at all depends on several factors: how much carbohydrate you currently eat in relation to how much you will be eating (the bigger the drop in carbs, the more likely the symptoms), and how sugar- or carb-addicted you are (the more addicted you are, the more likely you are to experience the symptoms). Any or all of these symptoms are totally normal as your brain and body start adapting to using fat as a fuel source rather than carbohydrate. For most people this isn't a simple switch: the machinery for doing so will require some biochemical re-orchestration to the default energy system that humans have run on for millennia. With extreme carb restriction, when there is no longer enough glucose to fuel the brain, the body switches fuel sources and starts supplying ketones to the brain – which, by the way, functions perfectly well on both. A ketone body is formed when fat is broken down in the body when it is being used for fuel. The presence of ketones in your blood indicates that you are burning fat as an exclusive fuel source (i.e., you are completely "fat adapted").

Quick tips

How to manage or alleviate these symptoms:

CHOOSE YOUR TIMING

I strongly suggest that you plan for the start of your LCHF journey in advance (particularly the more extreme the carb restriction). If you have a job that requires top-level thinking and attention, then it is best to start LCHF on a Thursday or Friday or while you're on holiday. It takes a couple of days to substantially reduce or deplete the body's glycogen (stored sugar) reserves. Then you can have the "down" couple of days over the weekend, and hopefully most of the symptoms will be gone by the start of the next week. It is critical during this phase that when you crave sweet things or carbs, you don't succumb. Treat it like detox or rehab – carb addiction can be as powerful as addiction to mainstream toxic drugs.

INCREASE YOUR SALT INTAKE

This is important. Whatever the level of carb restriction you decide on, you do need to have more salt to help manage some of the symptoms, particularly light-headedness and fatigue. During the early adaptation phase, as the body adjusts, water is lost from the body alongside the drop in carb storage (1 g carb is stored in the body together with 3 g water). Consequently, the electrolytes sodium and potassium experience some temporary imbalance, which can leave you feeling a little "off." With extreme carb restriction this is often called "keto-flu," as for a couple of days you just feel like staying in bed (hence the importance of timing). You will also probably be eating less processed food and thus less salt overall, which further stresses the importance of supplementing with salt during this time.

OH NO, NOT CONSTIPATION!

During early adaptation, this can sometimes happen. There are several things you can do to sort this out, including ensuring that you drink enough water/fluid and eat enough vegetables for fiber – but most importantly you need to eat enough fat. Sounds strange, I know, but usually upping the fat intake will solve this for most people. Another good reason to get over your fear of fat!

To help prevent or alleviate these symptoms, add half a teaspoon of salt to your existing food intake or consume 1-2 cups of broth each day (stock cubes mixed in water).

Got your level of carb restriction and your timing sorted out? Now all that's left is to get started . . . so read on.

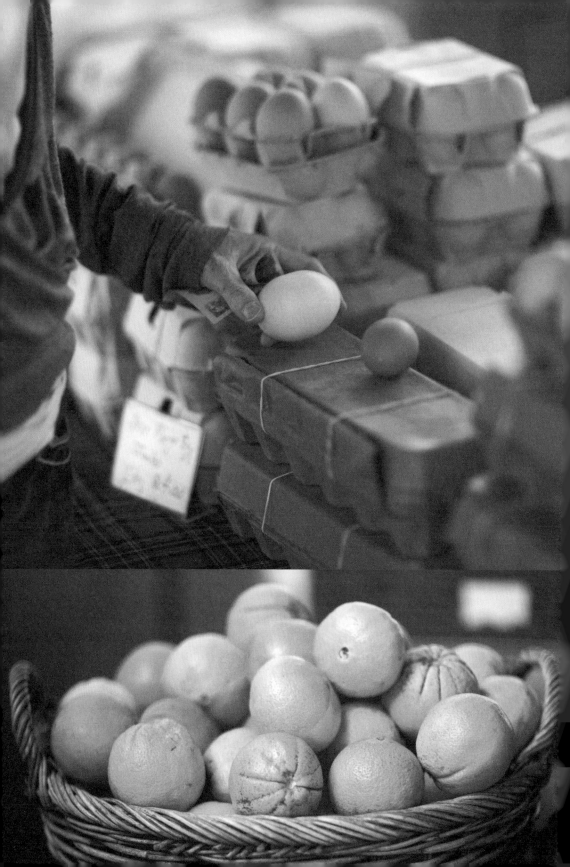

The 10 rules

The LCHF concept is essentially quite simple: if you truly eat only "whole foods," you will naturally end up eating less carbohydrate and more fat than you do in your current diet.

However, there are lots of extra snippets of information required to do LCHF effectively. I have summarized these for yowu into ten simple rules. Practiced regularly, these rules soon become habits – and before you know it you will be embracing this way of eating and thinking without second-guessing yourself. Here we go . . .

Go low "HI"

No, I'm not referring to the GI (Glycemic Index), but the Human Interference factor, a term coined by the Fat Professor himself. The HI factor is a scale indicating the extent to which a food has encountered human interference (HI) – in other words, the level of processing that food has been subjected to. On a scale of 1 to 10, 1 indicates the least interfered-with or processed food (low HI) and 10 indicates the most interfered-with or processed (high HI). Vegetables such as broccoli or cauliflower would have an HI factor of 1, and pasta or crackers would have an HI factor of 10. We find the HI factor a great way to view foods, assisting our decision making: if you ever get lost in the details of foods, consider their HI factor and choose predominantly low HI, unprocessed whole foods.

Cut the carbs (down . . . not out)

The foods we eat typically contain a wide range of nutrients, both macro (carbs, protein, and fat) and micro (vitamins and minerals), rather than one nutrient only. We can, however, largely classify foods into main macronutrient categories. For example, sugar, sugary drinks, honey, bread, cereals, noodles, rice, commercial crackers and granola bars, fruit, vegetables, milk, and yogurt all contain carbohydrate. That said, not all carbs are equal.

With LCHF eating, we want to ensure that good-quality carbs make up your daily allocation. In this sense, LCHF is about both quality and quantity. Let's go through the three different categories of carbohydrates. I like to describe them as "The Good," "The Bad," and "The Ugly."

Let's start with "The Good." Foods such as fruit, vegetables, dairy products, and legumes contain the best-quality carbs. While the actual carbs they provide are processed by the body in exactly the same way as refined sugar, these foods also provide a wide spectrum of beneficial nutrients such as fiber (from fruit, vegetables, and legumes), and calcium and protein (from dairy products). They are the least-processed carbs, have the lowest HI (Human Interference) factor, and hold a lot of water.

Remember, this is not NCHF (No-Carb, Healthy-Fat) but LCHF. Some carbs are intended; we just need to select the best-quality ones.

Secondly, let's explore "The Bad." Foods such as breads, cereals, pasta, noodles, rice, granola bars, and crackers are predominantly carbohydrate, but they also contain protein and fat. They too are handled in the same way in the body as refined sugar, but the difference here is that compared with whole foods they are low in nutrient density and are very processed. This label, "The Bad," is perhaps a little extreme, but hopefully you get the message. Maybe a better way to describe these foods is discretionary carbs.

Finally, "The Ugly." The worst of the carb bunch are refined carbs such as sugary drinks and sweets, and sugar itself, which is found in many, many foods. These foods typically provide nothing beneficial for the body and I consider them harmful; sugar has even been described as toxic. It's good to see the detrimental effects of sugar becoming universally recognized now; if these foods feature regularly in your diet, it's time to cut them out. They add nothing and will only make you unhealthy.

Avoiding the "ugly" carbs requires an appreciation of the many cunning places sugar hides in our food. This might surprise you. In fact, there are around a hundred different names for sugar, half of which I have never even heard of. Sugar goes under various pseudonyms on food labels – such as sucrose, lactose, maltose, galactose, fructose, maltodextrin, dextrose, xylose, and glucose, to name a few. There are also lots of other forms of sweetener that are supposedly better than sugar itself – see examples in the list opposite.

Despite the variety of names, your body knows that all of these are sugar and handles them in exactly the same manner as normal table sugar (or sucrose). So don't be fooled; your body won't be. Nutrition science is complex and can be very confusing for consumers, who are expected to decipher food labels and make the best decision. Where possible, selecting foods that don't have labels (i.e., whole foods) is an easy way to avoid the confusion.

COMMON SWEETENERS

- Honey
- Agave syrup/nectar
- Honey barley malt
- Molasses
- Caramel syrup
- Treacle
- Golden syrup
- Corn and brown rice syrup
- Beet, brown, raw, cane, date, demerara, superfine, and coconut sugar . . . to name just a few.

Virtuous vegetables

I cannot stress enough the importance of vegetables in the LCHF lifestyle. Removing processed, grain-based products from our diets means removing some fiber, vitamins, and minerals, so it is essential to increase your vegetable intake; substantially for some. I strongly recommend including vegetables multiple times over the course of the day, in meals and/or snacks. As with carbs in general, not all vegetables are created equal. We can separate them into two main categories: non-starchy vegetables and starchy vegetables.

The majority of non-starchy vegetables grow above ground. They provide lots of nutrients (such as vitamins and minerals), but very little carbohydrate. They include leafy greens (lettuce, spinach, kale, Swiss chard), broccoli, cauliflower, zucchini, carrots, celery, tomatoes, cucumbers, green beans, mushrooms, and onions. These vegetables can (and should) be included ad lib (which means as much as you want); there is no limit on them with moderate carb restriction. For extreme carb restriction (i.e., the ketogenic diet), pay closer attention to the amounts consumed, as even small amounts of carbs in lots of vegetables add up quickly.

Starchy vegetables include those growing below the ground. While they provide vitamins and minerals, along with these comes a lot of added carbohydrate. These vegetables include potatoes, sweet potatoes, parsnips, beets, squash, yam, taro, peas, and corn. It's not that you can't eat these vegetables, but instead a matter of including them less regularly and/or in smaller quantities than the non-starchy vegetables.

Your balance of starchy and non-starchy vegetables depends on your personal goal, the amount and type of activity you're doing, and the level of carb restriction you select. Potato and sweet potato are often consumed in large amounts in one sitting (e.g., in mashed potatoes) along with other starchy vegetables (in a "Sunday roast," for example), whereas beets or peas might be consumed in smaller portions in any one meal. Given that everyone is different, the best thing to do is to prioritize your carbs, choosing types to suit your level of restriction and the occasion for which they're being provided.

Make fat your friend

The number-one barrier to the successful implementation of a whole-food, *LCHF* lifestyle is the fear of fat. This is totally understandable after fifty years of being told (incorrectly) to eat as little fat as you can, particularly saturated fat. Not eating enough fat leads to two problems: you end up with either a low-carb, low-fat diet (which means not eating much at all and being left feeling hungry), or (most commonly) a low-carb, low-fat, high-protein diet (protein levels having been raised to help you feel full, and because you've got to eat something, right?). Overeating protein is a problem for one simple reason: excessive amounts of protein are metabolized by the liver into glucose – that's right, sugar! This is counterproductive and tantamount to eating high carb.

But how much fat and what type of fat?

How much fat you should eat is determined by two things: your overall goal and your total daily energy requirement. Energy requirements are different for everyone, dependent as they are on body size, body composition, and daily movement (be that incidental movement or formal exercise). Sadly, there is no "fat prescription" like there is for carbohydrate. My advice is to include as much or as little fat in each meal to allow you to feel full and to take you to the next main meal without feeling that you need a snack in between. Some trial and error is required with this: listen to your body to work out exactly what works for you.

As you know, our take on LCHF is Low-Carb, *Healthy*-Fat. The types of fat you should be eating are summarized here in our top ten "go to" fats or fat sources.

Olive oil

Rich in vegetable-based monounsaturated fat and antioxidants, olive oil and flavored olive oils are my top-quality cooking fats and a great way to increase the fat content of your salad and vegetable meals. I advocate making your own salad dressings rather

than buying commercial ones that contain cheap and processed industrial seed oils – see chef Craig's great examples on page 130. They really are quick and easy.

The most important thing about cooking with any oil is that the oil should not be heated to above its smoke point, which is the temperature at which an oil begins to break down, burn, and give food a bad taste. Olive oil can be used for cooking at high temperatures, but this depends on the quality of the oil itself, with the better-quality oils having higher smoke points. My best advice is to buy a good-quality olive oil (i.e., extra-virgin olive oil) if you want to use it for high-temperature cooking; otherwise, use other fats for cooking, as shown below.

Coconut oil

Due to its stable structure, this oil is also suitable for cooking foods at high temperatures. Coconut oil contains a lot of saturated fat, which in the context of our existing carb- and sugar-laden processed-food diet is problematic for health if consumed in large quantities. But in the context of LCHF, where you are eating whole, unprocessed foods, including saturated fat along with other types of fat (but not trans fats), coconut oil is fine. Use the deodorized version of coconut oil when cooking foods you don't want tainted with a coconut tang, and the non-deodorized version for making homemade grain-free granola to add a delicious coconut flavor.

Coconut products

Coconut cream or milk is an easy way to boost the fat intake of your breakfast, in a smoothie or poured over yogurt and grain-free granola. It's also perfect in a curry for a great evening meal (served on cauliflower rice – see Craig's recipe on page 154). Coconut flesh itself, chopped up into small chunks, also makes a great snack – and it's fun getting the coconut open!

Avocado

Highly nutritious and an extremely effective way to increase the fat content of a salad, avocados are a magnificent source of monounsaturated fat. They can also form the base of guacamole to use as a dip.

Macadamia nuts

Depending on how they are prepared, these can be 70-80 percent fat. They are so delicious that once you start eating them you sometimes can't stop; and while fat is good, you can still overdo it if you're not careful. Be wary of overeating macadamias, as it's easy to "go nuts on nuts."

Nut butter

Nut butters make a great dip for chopped vegetables, a spread on grain-free crackers, or an addition to smoothies for a little extra protein. Some great blends now exist, such as almond and cashew butter, or peanut butter blended with sunflower or pumpkin seeds. Check for no added sugar on peanut butter. Nut butters can be quite expensive, but are easily made yourself with a good, powerful blender.

Cheese

No need to choose the lowest fat cheese anymore – all cheese types are back on the menu, including delicious and often "stinky" blue vein, stringy mozzarella and strong Parmesan. They all provide a good amount of fat, as well as protein and calcium.

Cream

Plain cream, either poured or whipped, is a great way to turn a cup of berries into a filling and delicious meal or snack. Try frozen berries with thickened cream or mascarpone, creating an almost ice-cream-like consistency. Cream can also be added to a smoothie, casserole, or coffee, helping to keep you full.

Butter

Rich in the fat-soluble vitamins A, D, and K2, as well as a host of other compounds that are beneficial for health, butter is delicious to cook with. Melted, it adds a great taste poured over vegetables.

Fatty meat

That's right: there is no need anymore to look for the leanest cut of meat or trim the fat off before you cook or eat it. Crispy chicken skin and pork crackling can now be enjoyed, so eat them guilt-free! Arguably, it can even be good for you (see page 213 in Part 3: Unlocking the real science). Sausages are another great way to get some added fat, provided that you get good-quality ones from your butcher that aren't packed full of wheat and starchy fillers (as many of the supermarket varieties are).

Fats to avoid

Avoiding trans fats is a must. Trans fats are a type of unsaturated fat. Fortunately, because they are uncommon in nature and are created artificially, they are mostly found in packaged, processed bakery and confectionery-based items, and are therefore not such a problem with whole-food LCHF eating.

Despite what we've been told for years, there is now good evidence to suggest that we should also avoid the manufactured polyunsaturated seed oils such as canola, sunflower, soybean and rice bran oils. This is not so much about trans fats, but more about the level of processing required to manufacture these oils, and also about the inflammatory nature of their fatty-acid profile (i.e., lots of omega-6 fats, very little omega-3 fats – we want more omega-3s!). By removing these oils, we can reduce inflammation and improve health. Beware of supposed "healthy" products, such as nuts, olives, and canned fish, as they often have these cheap, processed seed oils added to them. Choose foods that are bathing in olive oil only.

5

Put protein in its place

Remember, LCHF does not call for a high-protein intake. While protein is a nutrient that helps you stay full, too much protein gets converted into glucose (or carbohydrate) in the body. If you overeat protein, you end up eating a higher-carb diet than you think you're eating, which defeats the purpose of going low carb.

Given that we still need some protein, however, how much is too much? Your unique protein requirement depends upon your body size and composition, age, stress levels, activity levels, the type of activity you do, and of course your goals. When doing LCHF, two key take-home messages apply.

Firstly, spread the protein in reasonably even proportions throughout the day to make sure that each meal has a protein and fat satiety combination.

Secondly, try not to exceed much beyond palm-sized servings of protein-based foods. As a guide, 100-120 g of meat, fish, or chicken (palm size) provides roughly 30-35 g of protein. In case you're wondering, the rest of the weight is made up of fat, connective tissue, water, and bone.

Mainstream requirements for protein intakes range from 0.8 g/kg of body weight for a sedentary individual (which I'm hoping you are not!) to 1.6-1.8 g/kg or a little more if you have muscle-growth needs. A common misconception is that athletes need a lot more protein than non-athletes, but in fact, their requirements are only a little greater, and easy to achieve from eating whole foods. Those of you trying to get into nutritional ketosis need to be a lot stricter with your protein intake. The required amount varies widely from person to person, but as a general rule I tend to set a threshold of somewhere around 1.5 g of protein per kg of your ideal body weight. This is not a lot, particularly if your body weight is at the lower end of the spectrum. It would be a definite cutback for most people. While you don't need to remain that strict if you are adopting the general LCHF principles, it still pays to be mindful of the amount of protein you eat.

A word on vegetarians and vegans

Vegetarians need to obtain their protein from vegetable protein sources, including beans and legumes, nuts and seeds, tofu and soy products. These foods tend to be two-thirds carbs and one-third protein (apart from the nuts and seeds, which vary more), making it a little more challenging for vegetarians to reduce carbs without compromising protein intake. This is just something to acknowledge, however – it can still be done. Those eating eggs and fish will find it easier. Vegans will find it more difficult, but can still follow the general concepts.

'If you overeat protein, you end up eating a higher-carb diet than you think you're eating, which defeats the purpose of going low carb.'

Eat on cue

The LCHF lifestyle does a beautiful job of allowing us to get in touch with our natural hunger and satiety (fullness) cues. Because both protein and fat provide us with that "satiety factor," including both in every meal helps us to gauge when we are satisfied during meal consumption.

Of course, we need to still be mindful that the rate at which we eat, and the settings in which we eat, influence our food intake. When we eat too fast, we fail to register our satiety feelings and can overeat. Eating in front of the TV or computer screen places less emphasis on the eating experience – rather than eating slowly and enjoying our meal in a more conscious way, food is consumed mindlessly. Studies have shown that regardless of meal composition, people tend to overeat when their attention is directed elsewhere.

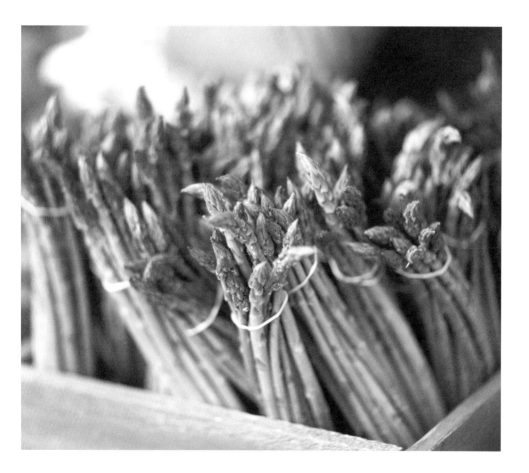

Sort your support

I don't encourage you to embark on LCHF alone. While it is a lifestyle change that's likely to be beneficial, you will need to get your support systems in place in order for it to become a reality (and be as smooth and easy a transition as possible). This includes support from family, friends, and work colleagues. The family is your first concern, as it is important to make this lifestyle change for them as well. While each family member might have different needs, the LCHF lifestyle and basic whole-food principles apply to everyone. If more carbohydrate is wanted by some family members, that's fine, so long as they select their carbs from whole-food sources. Ultimately, if the entire family embraces whole-food sources of carbohydrate, even with higher levels for some, everyone is better off than relying on processed foods.

What about your friends and work colleagues? You can only control what you can control, but I would strongly recommend that you at least tell people what you are doing, and explain your motivations. While they might not initially agree with your choice, seeing the delicious food and associated benefits are likely to prompt more questions, support, and perhaps even an inclination to try LCHF themselves. I hear stories about this happening repeatedly in my clinic.

Workplaces are notorious for regular birthday parties and gatherings that typically involve foods laden with sugar. If this is part of your three-meal "treat" (check out rule number 9) then fine, but if your colleagues are aware of what you are trying to achieve, then typically the coercion that goes along with these occasions will subside. Alternatively, introduce some healthier whole-food options to the mix so that you can participate without having to eat foods you choose not to eat.

Finally, you also need support from the places where you will be eating out. If you fancy a menu item but a part of it comes with carbs, all you need to do is ask for that component to be left out or changed. Many don't ask because they don't want to cause any inconvenience. Remember this: you are the paying customer, and as such you are allowed to request food you want to eat. Instead of ordering eggs on toast and leaving the toast on the side of the plate because you don't want to be an inconvenient customer, ask them to swap the toast for a side of creamed spinach, mushrooms, or broiled tomato. This means minimal wastage and ensures you get food you want to eat – plus more nutrients. Many cafés and restaurants are used to this and are happy to oblige. Over time, with enough people asking, café and restaurant menus will change to meet the low-carb demands of their customers. It's already happening.

'If your colleagues are aware of what you are trying to achieve, then typically the coercion that goes along with office parties will subside.'

Diligence, not effort

Diligent is how you should be viewing your LCHF lifestyle tasks of meal planning, shopping, storing, preparing, and cooking food, rather than effortful. LCHF eating is a lifestyle, not a "diet" or a "fad." Diligence is about consistency and mindfulness. Once you've got the principles and rules in your head, then ongoing, gentle policing of your actions is all that's required. Be diligent.

I don't believe there is any point in starting something to meet a specified goal and then stopping. That's a "diet"! We don't believe in diets; we are more interested in helping you see the sense and giving you the tools to assist with a change in mindset. Consider, for example, how you look after your teeth: you brush them each morning and night and you floss (hopefully) – which can seem like an effort, but you do it to preserve your teeth, which you understand are important to you.

"Dietary diligence" is just as important: every single cell in your body is dependent on what you put in your mouth. Make the attempt to look after your cells, and you're going to be looking after your health and the health of your family. Think about the activities required to make this work: a little bit of meal planning, grocery shopping, storage of groceries, preparation of meals. Instead of viewing these as tasks or an effort, flip your mindset and look at it as an opportunity – the opportunity to set up for a well-organized week ahead in food and promoting health. Making these processes into rituals helps them happen with greater reliability. For example, on Saturdays I go shopping to ensure that I have enough of the right food in the fridge, and on Sundays I prepare and cook for the week ahead. Remember: if you fail to prepare . . . you prepare to fail!

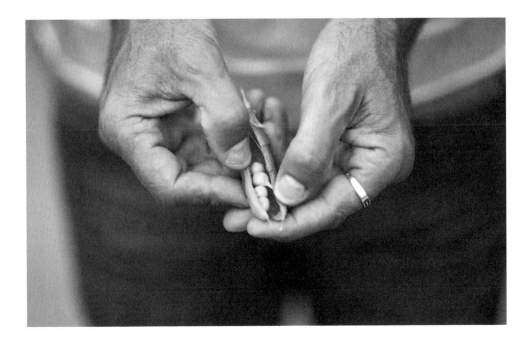

Adopt the three-meal rule

None of us is perfect – I'm not, and I certainly don't expect you to be. Experience has shown that being too restrictive about eating is not sustainable in the long term. We all need to "live a little." There will always be birthdays, anniversaries, work parties, holidays, and other social functions. To be expected to not indulge in some "LCHF-unfriendly" celebratory pleasures is unrealistic. Just make sure that the treats don't become too frequent, prompting old habits to creep back in. The "three-meal" rule is a good way to think about treats. It works like this: of the 21 meals in a week (three meals a day), achieving LCHF for 18 of these meals leaves three for you to choose what you want to eat. It could be sweet treats, carb-laden pizza or pasta, or some birthday cake. This is entirely up to you, but at least choose something you really like and want. And enjoy it! These three meals don't have to be scheduled in as "must have" cheat meals, but rather should be just dealt with as encountered. If you don't have any occasions like this for a couple of weeks, it is not a cue to save up all your treat meals to use in one week! It is rather about finding the balance between living LCHF most of the time and including non-LCHF friendly foods on the odd occasion.

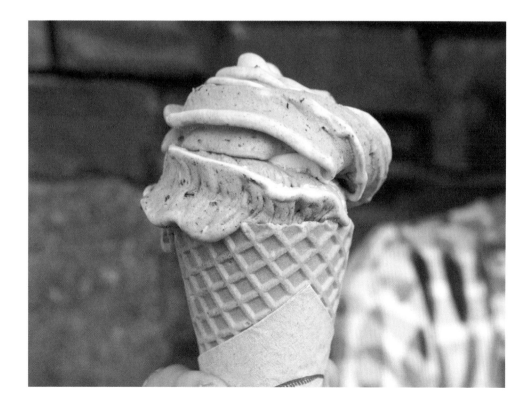

10

It's not just about the food

While LCHF is basically about food, the LCHF lifestyle is more holistic. We want to improve your health – so not smoking, reducing stress, eliminating environmental toxins, and ensuring optimal amounts of sleep, physical activity, and sun exposure are important. The word "optimal" is vital here, as too little or too much of these is no good (apart from smoking, of course, where abstinence is best).

The optimal amount of sleep, as shown by a recent study on 3,760 people over seven years, is 7.8 hours per night for men and 7.6 hours for women. The amount people sleep these days is less than in previous generations, largely due to our busy lives. Not getting enough sleep can have a negative health impact, including an increased risk of obesity and chronic disease. Sleep deprivation can stimulate appetite and cravings. It can also cause you to develop insulin resistance, which in turn means that you are less able to tolerate carbohydrate foods. Sleep needs to be made a priority for a healthy lifestyle. This might mean a little less TV, or switching off your light a little earlier than normal. However, too much sleep can have similar negative health effects, so it's that "optimal" amount of almost eight hours you are aiming for.

Physical activity (a.k.a. exercise) is an incredibly important component of optimal living. Like sleep, it is not about going for as long and hard as you possibly can. This places undue stress on the body, risks injury, and may have negative long-term effects. The optimal amount of physical activity varies from person to person. Ideally, make it regular, include activity to raise the heart rate to maintain or improve your cardiovascular fitness, and include some weight-bearing activity to keep bones and muscles in good shape. Finally, make it enjoyable to ensure that it is sustainable in the long term. Naturally, the amount and the intensity of your physical activity depends on your personal goals and situation.

Optimal sun exposure is another, often underestimated, contributor to good health. The sun's UVB rays enable the vitamin D generated by the body to be converted into its active form. Activated vitamin D is an important fat-soluble vitamin for health, and a deficiency in this vitamin can result in compromised bone health. We have been thoroughly alerted to the detrimental effects of spending too much time in the sun, but now we seem to have gone the other way and are getting too little sun exposure. This results in vitamin D deficiency for a small percentage of certain population groups. We need to aim for safe sun exposure to get that balance right. It's still important to slather on the sunscreen and cover up, but we also need to allow a little sun exposure. Get some sun, just don't get sunburned.

'Optimal sun exposure is another, often underestimated, contributor to good health.'

Getting set up

This is the start of your new life of whole food. A new start goes hand in hand with a clearing-out of your old life, which may include some bad habits and foods.

Once you have mastered the concept of being organized – not only for one week, but week in, week out – old habits are less likely to creep back in, and a successful sustainable lifestyle change for you and your family becomes far more likely.

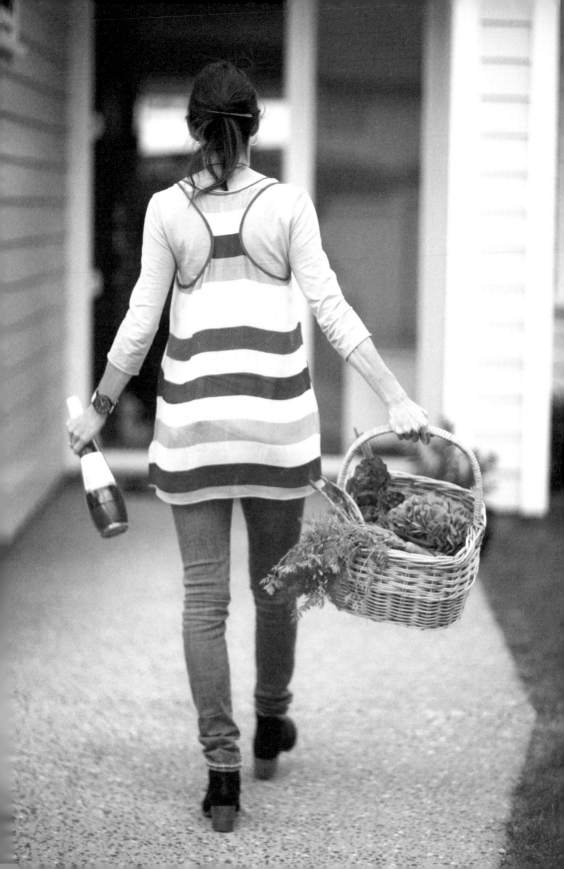

Clearing out and restocking

Embrace the kitchen concept "full fridge, empty pantry." Your new whole-food, LCHF life begins with a clean-out. Packaged foods, which you now view as high in carbohydrate, laden with sugar, and nutrient-poor, have no place in your house. They simply need to go. Throw them out or give them away. Not just out of sight (as in at the back of the pantry), but gone from the house itself. Your new kitchen set-up is going to be built around the "full fridge, empty pantry" concept. Some pantry essentials are required, but only those listed on the right.

Full fridge

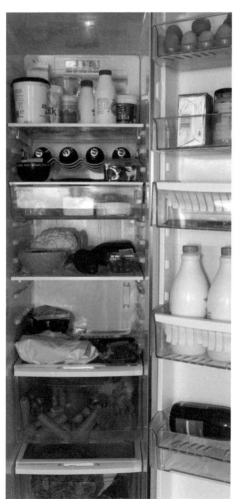

Empty pantry

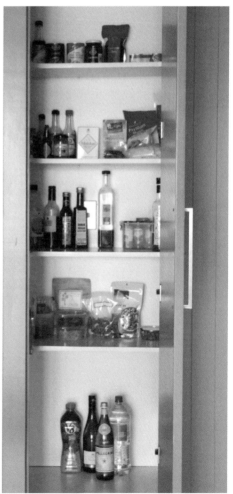

The fridge essentials

VEGETABLES

Choose a variety of different-colored vegetables. Always select seasonal vegetables.

- Greens: broccoli, kale, spinach, watercress, Swiss chard, celery, green beans, green onions, eggplant, Brussels sprouts, asparagus, zucchini, avocado, bok choy and other Asian greens
- Orange/reds: bell pepper, carrots
- Whites: cauliflower, mushrooms, fennel bulb

DAIRY PRODUCTS

- Cheese (any type, apart from the "plastic" and more heavily processed varieties)
- Full-fat milk, plain unsweetened Greek yogurt, butter, cream, sour cream

MEAT & OTHER PROTEINS

- Beef, lamb, chicken, pork, oxtail, venison, liver, kidneys
- Fish and shellfish
- Eggs

CONDIMENTS

- Mustard, pesto, relish, mayonnaise, aïoli, curry paste (always check the labels to ensure a low-sugar content, or better yet, make your own)

The freezer essentials

- Mixed berries
- Beef, chicken, lamb, fish, organ meat, prawns, marinara mix
- Vegetables

Leave space for frozen home-made meals.

The pantry essentials

HERBS & SPICES

- Salt (iodized rock salt and standard salt), cracked pepper, a selection of herbs and spices (e.g., turmeric, ground cumin, paprika, ground coriander, garam masala, curry powder, cinnamon, allspice), garlic, ginger

CANNED FOODS

- Salmon, tuna, sardines (in olive oil or brine only), whole or diced tomatoes, coconut milk/cream

Remove canned pasta and stir-fry sauces, canned fruit, creamed rice, baked beans. While you're at it, remove packaged items such as bread, noodles/pasta, rice, couscous, orzo, etc.

CONDIMENTS

Set yourself up with a variety of good oils. This can be an expensive initial set-up, but they will last as you will be using them interchangeably.

- Olive oil, avocado and other flavored oils, coconut oil, balsamic vinegar, Tabasco sauce, Worcestershire sauce, soy sauce, oyster sauce, tamari (gluten-free soy sauce), stock (cubes or liquid)

Remove heavily processed seed oils such as canola, sunflower, soybean, and rice bran oil, and sugary sauces such as sweet chili and tomato sauce/ketchup.

NUTS & SEEDS

- Raw almonds, cashews, Brazil nuts, walnuts, pine nuts, macadamias, pumpkin seeds/pepitas, sunflower seeds, chia seeds, flaxseed; nut butters – peanut (with no added sugar), almond, or cashew

Remove crackers, granola bars, breakfast cereals, oats.

BAKING & TREAT ITEMS

- Almond flour/meal, coconut flour, dark chocolate (70 percent cocoa or higher), baking soda, baking powder, xylitol or stevia

MISCELLANEOUS

- Desiccated coconut or coconut threads, psyllium husk

VEGETABLES

- Onions, shallots, small amounts of sweet potato, potato, beet, hard-shelled squash/pumpkin, parsnip

OTHER

- Storage containers. These will be very handy for storing vegetables in the fridge, preserving their freshness and fridge life.

Meal planning

My number-one tip for making the whole-food LCHF lifestyle sustainable is to make it easy for yourself. How do you do this? Simple: get organized!

Grocery shopping is often classed as a chore rather than a pleasant experience. Remember my tip about making LCHF sustainable? That's right, it's all about making it easy for yourself in the supermarket, produce market, or butcher shop. Making a shopping list would be the simple answer to a smoother shopping experience, but I want you to go back one step further. It is worth spending the time putting some thought and effort into meal planning and then creating your list.

Once you are in the habit of doing this, you will enjoy the many benefits of the LCHF lifestyle, including:

- A less stressful shopping experience.
- A less expensive weekly grocery bill.
- Buying fewer "extra things" that aren't meant to be in your shopping cart or basket.
- Saving time and gas money on extra mid-week trips.
- Saving money and your health by not resorting to takeout or last-minute packaged food.
- Less "package" waste, and being more environmentally friendly.

Allow some flexibility in your weekly menu to keep it realistic. For example, take advantage of special food offers – if you had planned to make a nice lasagne with eggplant as your "pasta" sheets, but eggplant is expensive and zucchini are on special, buy zucchini instead. Factor in a takeout meal and think about how you can make it LCHF-friendly (e.g., Thai or Indian takeout served with some home-made cauliflower rice you have in the fridge from earlier that week), or have a night out (follow our "Tips for eating out" guide on page 77). You could also involve your family (or housemates) in the process of planning meals to make it more fun and acceptable. Use a plan like the one on page 62 to help make your list.

There's nothing more satisfying than eating from your own herb and veggie garden.

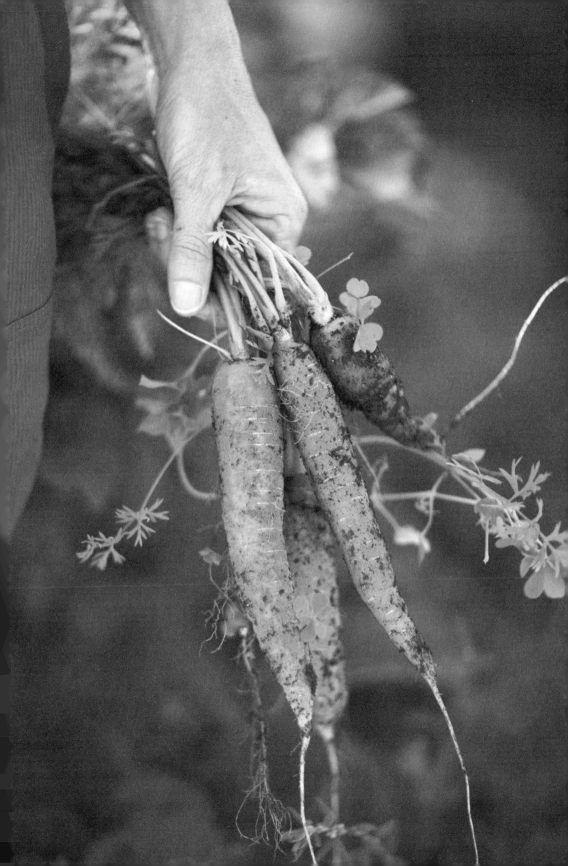

Weekly meal planner and shopping list example

	Breakfast	Lunch	Dinner
Monday	Green smoothie	Leftovers from Sunday roast	Roast chicken with cauliflower cheese and green vegetables
Tuesday	Green smoothie	Chicken salad	Roasted salmon with stir-fried broccoli and bok choy
Wednesday	Fruit, yogurt, granola	Tinned salmon salad	Beef and liver meatballs with vegetables
Thursday	Fruit, yogurt, granola	Leftover meatballs in salad	Cold-smoked salmon on salad
Friday	Fruit, yogurt, granola	Leftovers in salad	Thai takeout with cauliflower rice
Saturday	Bacon, eggs, vegetables	Tuna salad	Friends for dinner: crispy pork belly with stir-fried vegetables
Sunday	Bacon, eggs, vegetables	Chicken salad	Roast lamb with vegetables
Snacks	Fruit, mixed nuts, dried meat, coconut flesh, boiled eggs, chopped veggies		

Shopping list

- **Meats:** large chicken, beef, bacon, liver, pork belly, lamb, fresh and cold-smoked salmon, tuna . . .
- **Fruit:** berries (fresh and frozen), kiwifruit . . .
- **Vegetables:** cauliflower, spinach, tomato, cucumber, bell pepper, broccoli, bok choy . . .
- **Other:** coconut, nuts, eggs, yogurt . . .

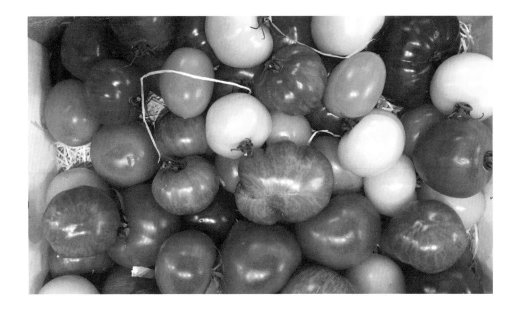

Shopping and stocking

Plan at least one regular weekly food shop, and try to do it when you are not rushing (if that's possible these days). Shopping at the supermarket is over-rated, as 90 percent of all the products on the shelves are packaged and processed. What's more, the cheaper and more "unhealthy" products positioned at eye-level are designed to lure you in. If you're shopping with young children this can be disastrous with so many temptations and "no" items risking additional drama.

Make it easier for yourself by shopping at a local fruit-and-vegetable store and butcher shop (it will be cheaper as well). You can pretty much get everything you need from these two shops. Non-perishables can still come from the supermarket. Consider ordering online. If the hassle of shopping at several places instead of one is overwhelming, then stick to shopping around the edges of the supermarket without being tempted to venture down the middle aisles. There might be some pantry set-up foods you need, such as canned fish and coconut cream, but unless it's on the list and planned for, don't deviate. Be diligent, remember!

Now, you might think that once you've shopped you can shove the produce in the fridge and pantry and get on with the rest of your day's activities . . . but not so fast! Another part of this "making it easy for yourself" journey is to spend a bit of time organizing your fridge. Time to use those storage containers I mentioned when I talked about pantry essentials.

Wash your vegetables and place them in storage containers, including your leafy green lettuce or spinach (remove it from the package it comes in). Chop or break your cauliflower and broccoli into florets before storing them. If you make the time to do this, your vegetables will remain fresh for 2–3 days longer, plus you can enjoy opening your fridge and basking in its "order." Trust me on this one – take pride in the orderly appearance of your fridge contents. Your food will look more appetizing and you'll quickly be able to identify some convenient whole-food options for snacks when you open it. There will also be minimal wastage, another great way to save your hard-earned money.

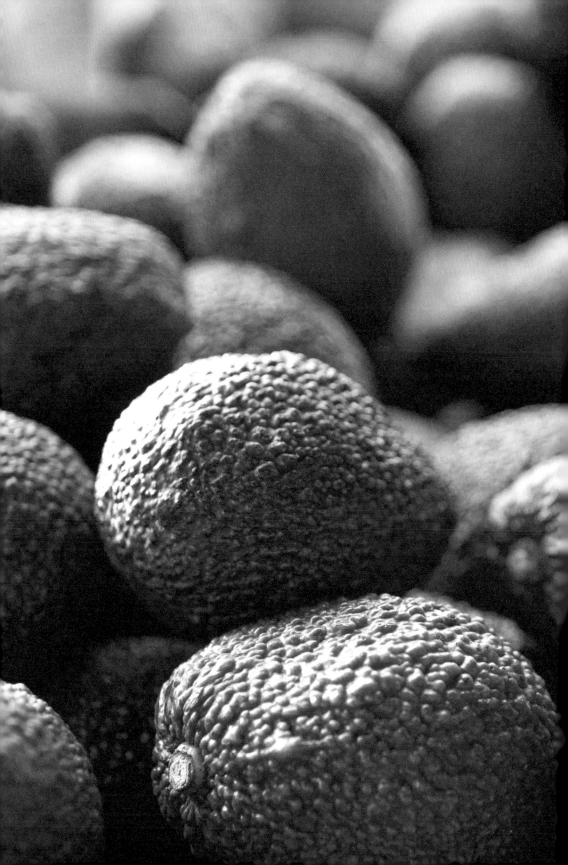

What's in, what's out

Over the next few pages, I present you with lists of foods that are in, foods that are out, and foods that are in . . . sometimes.

I like to use this quick guide to using these lists:

FOODS THAT ARE IN	FOODS THAT ARE IN, SOMETIMES	FOODS THAT ARE OUT
Yes!	Maybe . . .	No.

All items are listed in categories in alphabetical order, rather than in order of benefit. Each category of food and beverage is presented with its unique serving size, followed by the amount of carbohydrate it contains. There are always going to be "gray areas," and it is natural to be a little confused about the place, frequency, or amount of certain foods and beverages that you include. These decisions are all based on your personal level of carb restriction and the progress you are making towards achieving your goals. While it's not perfect, or exhaustive, it's a good guide to get you started.

WHAT SHOULD I EAT? YES!

- Good-quality carbs from whole foods that are minimally processed, such as vegetables (lots of non-starchy ones), fruit, dairy products, and the occasional legume.

- Protein from minimally processed meat, fish, chicken, eggs, dairy, nuts, and seeds.

- Fat from whole, minimally processed plants and animal sources, including avocado, olive oil, nuts, fatty fish, dairy products, coconut products, and fat/skin on meat and poultry.

WHAT SHOULD I BE CAUTIOUS OF? MAYBE . . .

- Processed meats and cheese.

- Naturally or artificially sweetened foods and drinks and packaged "low-carb" bars.

- Legumes, large quantities of starchy vegetables, and high-sugar fruits.

WHAT SHOULDN'T I EAT? NO.

- Refined and processed junk foods containing sugar.

- Refined, nutrient-poor, packaged carbohydrate-rich foods, including most grains, such as breads, cereals, pasta, rice, granola bars, and crackers.

Vegetables (1 serving = ½ cup, or as stated)

Yes!	Maybe . . .	No.
Non-starchy, fresh or frozen	**Starchy, fresh or frozen**	Any vegetable deep-fried in highly processed vegetable oils
Alfalfa sprouts, raw (0.1 g)	Corn on the cob, cooked (1 small or ½ cup kernels = 14.8 g)	
Artichoke hearts, cooked (1.1 g)	Pumpkin, cooked (9.9 g)	
Asparagus, cooked (1.6 g)	Parsnip, cooked (9.7 g)	
Avocado (0.6 g)	Potato, cooked (10.8 g)	
Beans, green, cooked (1.9 g)	Squash - buttercup, cooked (20.0 g)	
Beets, cooked (5.6 g)	Sweet potato, cooked (13.7 g)	
Belgian endive, 1 head, raw (2.1 g)	Taro, cooked (18.7 g)	
Bell pepper - red, raw (3.2 g)	Yam, cooked (19.5 g)	
Bell pepper - green, raw (1.2 g)		
Broccoli, cooked (0.1 g)		
Brussels sprouts, cooked (1.0 g)		
Bok choy, cooked (0.4 g)		
Butternut, cooked (7.0 g)		
Cabbage, cooked (1.1 g)		
Cabbage, napa, cooked (0.8 g)		
Carrot, raw (2.3 g)		
Cauliflower, cooked (1.8 g)		
Celery root, cooked (1.6 g)		
Celery, raw (1.8 g)		
Chives, raw (0.7 g)		
Cucumber, raw (1.3 g)		
Eggplant, cooked (1.1 g)		
Endive, raw (1.3 g)		
Fennel, raw (0.6 g)		
Garlic (1 clove = 0.5 g)		
Green onion, 1 raw (1.5 g)		
Herbs and spices - trace		
Kale, cooked (3.0 g)		
Kohlrabi, raw (2.8 g)		
Leek, cooked (3.2 g)		
Lettuce, raw (0.4 g)		
Mushroom, raw (0.1 g)		
Okra, raw (1.2 g)		
Olives (1.3 g)		
Onion, cooked (3.0 g)		
Peas, cooked (5.9 g)		
Radish, raw (1.6 g)		
Spinach, cooked (1.3 g)		
Snap peas, raw (7.1 g)		
Swiss chard, cooked (2.4 g)		
Tomato, raw (2.6 g)		
Turnip, cooked (1.4 g)		
Watercress, raw (0.04 g)		
Zucchini, cooked (1.0 g)		

Figures in parentheses show grams of carbohydrate per serving.

Fruit (1 serving = 1 medium piece, or as stated)

Yes!	Maybe ...	No.
Apple (13.0 g) Apricot, fresh (4.6 g) Avocado, ½ (0.5 g) Berries, mixed (frozen or fresh), ½ cup (4.5 g) Cherry, fresh, ½ cup (10.5 g) Coconut, fresh, ½ cup (1. 7g) Feijoa (1.7 g) Fig, fresh (4.8 g) Grapes, ½ cup (13.2 g) Grapefruit (11.8 g) Kiwifruit (8.0 g) Lemon, 1 small (10.0 g) Lime, 1 small (9.0 g) Mandarin (8.5 g) Mango, ½ cup (12.9 g) Melon, ½ cup (4.4 g) Nectarine (11.2 g) Orange (11.0 g) Papaya/pawpaw (5.1 g) Peach (9 g) Pear (19 g) Pineapple, ½ cup (9.3 g) Plum (6 g) Pomegranate, juice, ½ cup (15.1 g) Tamarillo (2.3 g) Watermelon, 1 slice (10.9 g)	Banana (31 g) Fruit, canned in juice, drained – e.g., ½ cup canned peaches (9.6 g)	Any fruit with sugar coating or deep-fried with highly processed vegetable oils (e.g., toffee apples, deep-fried bananas) Fruit, canned in juice, not drained, ½ cup (12.4 g) Fruit, canned in syrup, drained, ½ cup (13 g) Fruit, canned in syrup, not drained, ½ cup (28.9 g) Dried fruit, mixed, ½ cup (59 g)

Figures in parentheses show grams of carbohydrate per serving.

Animal-protein sources

Yes!	Maybe ...	No.
Eggs Fish: all species Good-quality bacon and sausages from any type of meat (no gluten or lactose fillers) Organ meats: liver, kidney, heart Poultry: any cuts or pieces of chicken, duck, pheasant, turkey (save the carcass/bones to make a bone broth) Red meat: all types, any cuts – beef, lamb, pork, ham, venison, veal, goat Seafood: mussels, clams, prawns, crayfish, scallops, abalone	Crumbed meats: frozen, crumbed fish fillets, fish cakes Cured/pickled/smoked meats and fish Lesser-quality processed meats: bacon, ham, salami/pepperoni, chorizo, other sausages	Highly processed/deep-fried meats (e.g., chicken nuggets/canned Spam)

All these foods have minimal, if any, carbohydrate in them, therefore no values have been listed.

Dairy (1 serving = ½ cup, or as stated)

Yes!	Maybe ...	No.
Butter (trace) Cheese, any type (trace) Cream (3.5 g) Crème fraîche (3.1 g) Milk, full fat/raw* (5.7 g) Sour cream (3.3 g) Yogurt, plain, unsweetened, full fat (3-8 g)	Cheese, processed (trace) Goat milk (5.4 g) Yogurt, plain, low fat, unsweetened (5.3 g) Yogurt, fruit, low fat (4.7 g)	Flavored milk (12.3 g) Ice cream (21-26 g) Yogurt, frozen (18 g) Yogurt, fruit/plain, low fat, sweetened (11-17g)

Figures in brackets show grams of carbohydrate per serving.
* Please note that if you are pregnant it is generally recommended to avoid unpasteurized (raw) milk.

Non-dairy (1 serving = ½ cup, or as stated)

Yes!	Maybe ...	No.
Coconut cream (3-5 g) Coconut milk (1-3 g) Unsweetened almond milk (0.4 g)	Rice milk (5.5 g) Soy milk (4.7 g)	Non-dairy creamer, 1 tsp (1 g) **

Figures in brackets show grams of carbohydrate per serving.
** Non-dairy creamer might be low in carbs, but it is made up of many processed and unhealthy non-food ingredients.

Nuts, seeds, and legumes* (1 serving = ½ cup, or as stated)

Yes!	Maybe . . .	No.
Almonds, raw (5.0 g) Brazil nuts, raw (2.9 g) Cashews, raw (13.0 g) Chia seeds, 1 Tbsp (6 g) Flaxseed, 1 Tbsp (0.5 g) Lima beans, cooked (1.4 g) Macadamia nuts, raw (3.2 g) Mung beans, raw, sprouted (3.2 g) Nut butter, 1 Tbsp (0.5-4 g) Pecans, raw (11.0 g) Pine nuts, raw (10.6 g) Pistachios, raw (8.9 g) Pumpkin seeds/pepitas, 1 Tbsp (1.6 g) Sesame seeds, 1 Tbsp (0.7 g) Sunflower seeds, 1 Tbsp (0.6 g) Walnuts, raw (2.3 g)	Black beans, cooked (13.4 g) Edamame/soy beans, cooked (7.5 g) Kidney beans, cooked (13.1 g) Navy beans, cooked (13.7 g) Lentils, cooked (10-13 g) Peanuts (6.2 g) Tofu, cooked (0.7 g)	Processed seed-based oils: sunflower, grapeseed, safflower, sesame Adzuki beans, cooked (24.5 g) Chickpeas, cooked (23.3 g) Pearl barley, cooked (20.7 g) Split peas, cooked (21.6 g)

Figures in brackets show grams of carbohydrate per serving.
* Legumes vary widely in their carb content; some are very high, so watch your portions.

Fats and oils

Yes!	Maybe . . .	No.
Avocado oil Butter Coconut oil Duck fat Lard Macadamia/other nut-based oil Olive oil	Hemp oil Peanut oil Sesame oil	Highly processed vegetable oils: canola, sunflower, rice-bran, soybean, corn, grapeseed, safflower, palm (environmental reasons) Margarine

All these foods have minimal, if any, carbohydrate in them, therefore no values have been listed.

Condiments, sauces and dressings* (1 serving = 1 tablespoon, or as stated)

Yes!	Maybe ...	No.
Aïoli, olive oil-based (1.1 g) Coconut milk/cream, ½ cup (2-3g) Curry paste (1.0 g) Fish sauce (0.8 g) Lemon/lime juice (0.3 g) Mayonnaise, olive oil-based, low sugar (0.2-3 g) Mustard (1.7 g) Oyster sauce (1.2 g) Pesto (0.7 g) Salad dressings made from good oils (see previous page) and vinegar Tamari (gluten-free soy sauce, 1.2 g) Tahini (0.2 g) Vinegars (0.1 g) Wasabi/horseradish sauce (1.7 g) Worcestershire sauce (3.1 g)	Commercial, high-sugar mayonnaise or aïoli that contains processed vegetable oils (see previous page) Chutney (6.3 g) Hummus (1-3 g) Salsa (1-7 g) Tomato relish (2-7 g) Tomato sauce, commercial (4 g)	Honey (16.5 g) Mint jelly (10 g) Pasta sauce, 1 cup (26 g) Syrup (11.4 g)

Figures in brackets show grams of carbohydrate per serving.

* A word on dressings. While many dressings and sauces are low in carbs (e.g., blue cheese, Caesar, ranch, French, Italian, etc . . .), store-bought varieties are often made with processed vegetable oils such as canola and sunflower oil. Try to find some that have olive oil only, or make your own.

Beverages (1 serving = 200 ml or 1 small cup)

Yes!	Maybe ...	No.
Coffee, brewed (0.8 g) Tea (0 g) Water, still or sparkling (0 g)	Diet drinks (0 g) Diet soda (0 g)	Cordial, concentrate, syrup, 2 Tbsp (17.5 g) Energy drinks (21.4 g) Flavored milk (19.7 g) Fruit juice (16-23 g) Soft drinks (22.5 g)

Figures in brackets show grams of carbohydrate per serving.

Alcohol** (1 serving = ½ cup, or as stated)

Yes!	Maybe ...	No.
Red/white wine, 1 glass, 100 ml (0-2.6 g) Spirits (whiskey, vodka, rum), 30 ml (0 g)	Beer, one 340-ml bottle (10-15 g) Cider, one 33- ml bottle (8.3 g)	

Figures in brackets show grams of carbohydrate per serving.

** Remember, alcohol is a toxin and a source of empty calories, so keep overall intake low in general.

Confectionery* (serving size as stated)

Yes!	Maybe . . .	No.
Dark chocolate: 55 percent cocoa, 2 squares, 20 g (1–10 g) Dark chocolate: 70 percent cocoa, 2 squares, 20 g (7–9 g) Dark chocolate: 85 percent cocoa, 2 squares, 20 g (5–8 g) Dark chocolate: 90 percent cocoa, 2 squares, 20 g (4–6 g)	Chocolate: dairy milk or other variety, 2 squares, 20 g (11–15 g) Sugar-free chewing gum (0 g)	Candy, e.g., 10 small jellybeans (10.3 g); 2 jelly snakes (40 g)

Figures in brackets show grams of carbohydrate per serving.
* Confectionery items are all high in sugar; part of embracing the LCHF lifestyle is about altering the "sweet" palate, so limit overall intake.

Sweeteners

Yes!	Maybe . . .	No.
	Natural sweeteners: stevia, Natvia, Xylitol	Artificial sweeteners: Equal, Sucaryl, Sugromax, Splenda

All sweeteners have minimal, if any, carbohydrate in them, therefore no values have been listed.

Miscellaneous

Yes!	Maybe . . .	No.
Japanese Konjac noodles (carb-free, made from an Asian fibrous vegetable), ½ cup (1 g)	Carb-free protein bars, 1 bar (4–6 g); watch for hidden carbs	Food made with highly processed vegetable oils

Figures in brackets show grams of carbohydrate per serving.

Need a nibble?

You'll pretty much kiss goodbye to snacking on LCHF because you'll feel fuller and won't get hunger pangs between meals, but there will be occasions where you might find you need a smaller meal.

The concept of snacking on LCHF is an interesting one, as I've found that making the switch to this way of eating pretty much removes the desire for snacks between meals. The fat and protein at each meal keeps you satiated. However, I acknowledge there might be times when snacks are appropriate. The traditional "three meals a day" style of eating might not work for you every day, particularly on weekends, and you might prefer a couple of smaller snacks instead. As long as you obtain enough nutrients from whole-food sources, how often and when you eat should largely be guided by how you feel and your personal circumstances. Snacks are often useful in the following situations: when traveling and available meal options are not "LCHF-friendly"; if your main meal doesn't contain enough fat or protein and you feel hungry a few hours later; or if you require a recovery meal after a hard workout and it's not yet time to eat a main meal. Remember, with LCHF eating, to let yourself be guided by your hunger cues, and make sure you are eating out of need, rather than out of boredom, habit, or dehydration. Over the page are some recommended snack options.

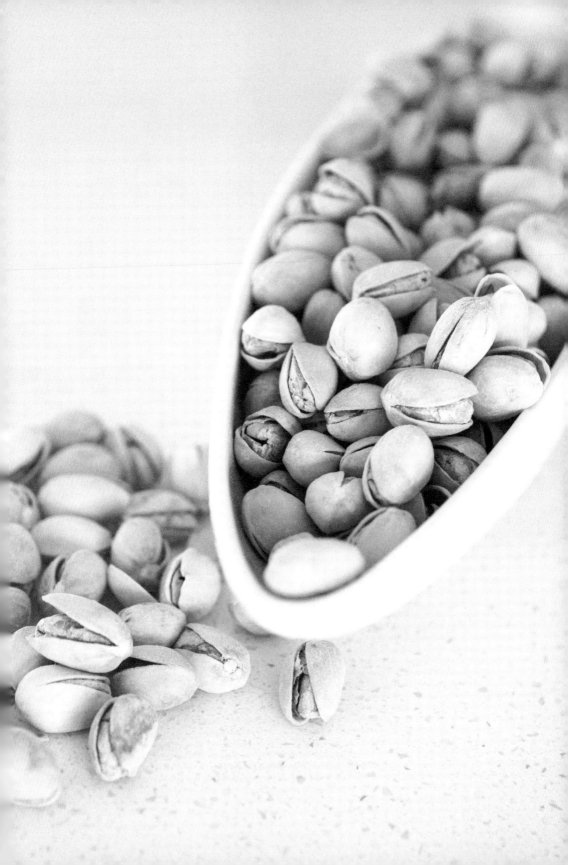

Your snacking chart

Fill a gap with any of these "LCHF-friendly" options.

Nuts

A variety of nuts is best for a range of nutrients. But do remember – don't "go nuts on nuts." They're easy to eat and the energy adds up, so watch your portions.

Eggs

Be prepared for your busy week ahead. Boil some eggs or make some quiche muffins when you have a bit more time on a weekend (see Craig's recipe on page 98), rather than stressing out during the mid-week chaos.

Veggies

Dip some sliced carrots, bell pepper, cauliflower, radish, or celery in guacamole, hummus, almond butter, or cream cheese.

Crackers

Enjoy Craig's amazing low-carb cracker recipe on page 172, or use cucumber rounds as a "cracker" base. Top with cheese, salmon, avocado, or Craig's nutrient-rich Chicken Liver Pâté (page 174).

Leftovers

If dinner was "LCHF-friendly," leftovers will make a perfect snack (chicken drumsticks, sausages, salad, veggies, etc.). It's not rocket science!

Coconut

Coconut flesh or "bombs" (desiccated coconut blended to a paste-like consistency, poured into molds or ice-cube trays, left to set in the fridge, and then stored in the cupboard) are a good way to increase your fat without adding protein. You might need a lesson in coconut cracking!

Dried meat

Bresaola, jerky, salami, and other dried meats. These foods are somewhat processed, so include occasionally rather than daily. Choose the least-processed versions you can find.

Berries & yogurt or cream

You can use any fruit you like – but berries have the lowest carb content and the greatest nutrient profile. Top with plain, unsweetened Greek yogurt or cream.

Cheese

Whether it's a mini Babybel, cubes of cheddar, salty halloumi, or a hunk of Camembert, cheese is where it's at as a snack. Portion size does count, though, as cheese can cause an insulin spike if eaten in large amounts – keep intake to around a matchbox size (30 g) each time you eat some.

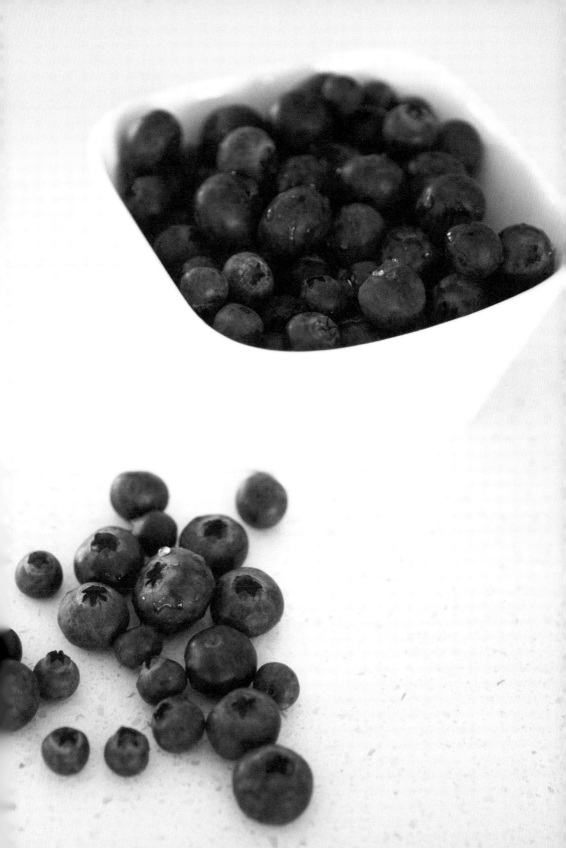

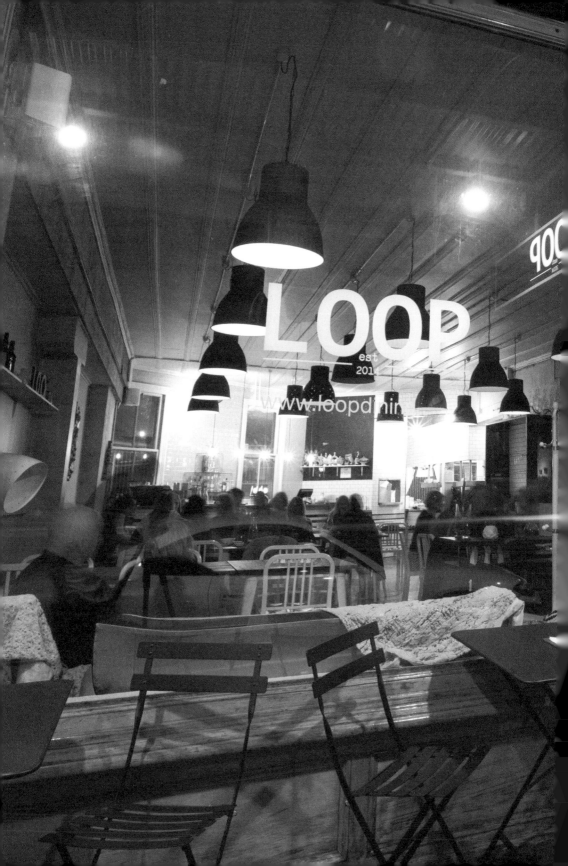

Tips for eating out

What the Fat? contains delicious recipes for home cooking, but as we're eating out a lot more these days, it pays to be prepared. Dining out on LCHF is not nearly as challenging as you might think. Most places (aside from big burger chains, pizza joints, and local bakeries) have some good-quality, "LCHF-friendly" options. Eating out does mean you lose a little control. By this, I mean you don't know what oils are being used to cook your food – but hey, there is only so much you can do.

01 DO YOUR HOMEWORK
Get to know where carbs are hiding in foods. Once you have this figured out, you will be armed to make the best selections.

02 JUST ASK!
Remember, you are the paying customer. You ask, you receive, it's as simple as that. The days of feeling embarrassed about saying "No bread, thank you" or "Can I please have some veggies instead of rice? are well and truly over. You will be surprised at how accommodating chefs are. Don't be shy, just ask!

Restaurant/café-style eating

Whatever and wherever you choose to eat, be it local cuisine, food from the East, or food from the West, you will always be able to find something you can enjoy.

Out for breakfast?
Go for eggs (any style), veggies (e.g., creamy mushrooms, tomato, spinach), liver, bacon, and sausage dishes. Enjoy smoothies made with coconut cream or regular cream. Nut-based granolas with natural yogurt and berries can be good, too, but watch for added honey, oats, and dried fruit. Ask for the toast to be held back. Ask to swap the hash browns for a broiled tomato or some spinach. Ask for the honey to be held back or swapped for cream.

Out for lunch or brunch?
Go for veggie-packed salads with olive oil-based dressings, creamy soups, and traditional "main meals" of protein (i.e., meat, fish, chicken, pork) with veggies or salad. Ordering a breakfast item for lunch (such as the ones listed above) is also a great option. Ask for the salad noodles to be held back. Ask for the croutons to be held back. Ask to swap the sugary salad dressing for olive oil and balsamic.

Out for dinner?
Go for a main meal of protein with veggies or salad. Our personal favorites include lamb shanks (Caryn), pork belly (Grant) and fresh fish (Craig) with veggies and/or salad. Ask for the burger bun to be held back, replacing it with romaine lettuce. Ask to swap the rice or mashed potato for salad or veggies. Ask to swap the sweet sauce for a creamy mushroom or pepper sauce. For dessert, you have three choices. One: just don't order any. Two: order your best low-carb option, such as a cheese board without the crackers. Three: use the "three-meal rule" (see page 54 for more on this) and really enjoy whatever it is you order, knowing that it's a treat occasion and treats are rare.

Eating on the run

If you're out and about and you need to eat but your options are limited, don't use up one of your three treat meals on junk food from the service station or sub-standard bakery food that leaves you feeling less than average and disappointed in yourself. No matter where you are, there are usually a range of options that will keep you on track.

24/7 convenience stores or service stations

Packets of plain mixed nuts, cans of tuna, fruit, water, tea or coffee with a dash of full-fat milk or cream (no sugar).

TIP: *Avoid pre-packaged meals with noodles or rice, and honey-roasted peanuts.*

Supermarkets

Fresh vegetables, fruit, raw mixed nuts, beef jerky, unsweetened natural yogurt, cheese, olives in brine or olive oil, canned fish, cold meats.

TIP: *Be careful with pre-made salads and hot, pre-roasted chickens, as they can often be prepared with processed vegetable oils and/or sugar-laden mayonnaise.*

Juice bars

Smoothies with unsweetened natural yogurt, coconut cream, cream, fruit; vegetable juices.

TIP: *Be careful with fruit-only drinks, as the natural sugar adds up.*

Bakery or café

Baseless quiche, fruit, tea or coffee with a dash of full-fat milk or cream (no sugar).

TIP: *Turn around, walk out of there, and go and find some good-quality food elsewhere!*

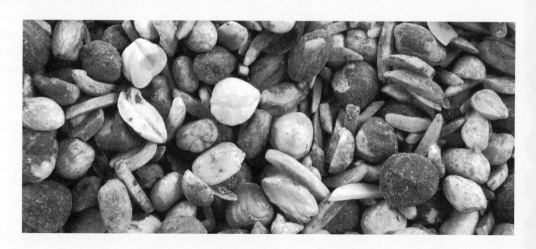

Facing fast food/takeout

There are two major types: big-chain fast food and small-chain fast food and cafés. The best option is to avoid the big chains entirely. Most traditional chains use poor-quality oils in cooking and lots of added sugar, making it hard to find an "LCHF-friendly" choice. At small chains, whether they're in town, at an airport, or out in the country, there are always good options to choose from. Some examples are listed below.

Big-chain fast food

McDonald's, KFC, Burger King
- Low-carb burger (no bun) with either grilled chicken or beef patty
- Grilled chicken and salad
- Scrambled eggs without a bun or toast
- Water, tea, or coffee with a dash of full-fat milk or cream

Small-chain fast food

Salad bars or designer sandwich places (e.g., Subway)
- Select your own salads: vegetables (mostly non-starchy), add protein (meat, fish, chicken, egg), add fat (avocado, cheese); pre-packaged Greek salad
- Ready-made meals with chicken/fish/meat with vegetables
- Fruit salad with unsweetened natural yogurt
- Scrambled eggs with veggies or salad

Gourmet burger joints
- Some places offer burgers with no bun, wrapped in lettuce instead

Japanese
- Sashimi (raw fish), seaweed salads, grilled chicken/beef with veggies (donburi), miso soup; avoid the noodles and rice

Takeout tips

Choose	Avoid
✓ Whole foods	✗ Bread
✓ Vegetables	✗ Pita
✓ Salad	✗ Wraps
✓ Fruit	✗ Croissants
✓ Meat	✗ Muffins
✓ Fish	✗ Pastry
✓ Chicken	✗ Pancakes
✓ Eggs	✗ Rice
✓ Nuts	✗ Noodle- or couscous-based salads
✓ Seeds	
✓ Water	✗ Ready-made meals
✓ Tea or coffee with a dash of full-fat milk or cream (no sugar)	✗ Fries
	✗ Muesli
	✗ Cake
	✗ Sugary drinks

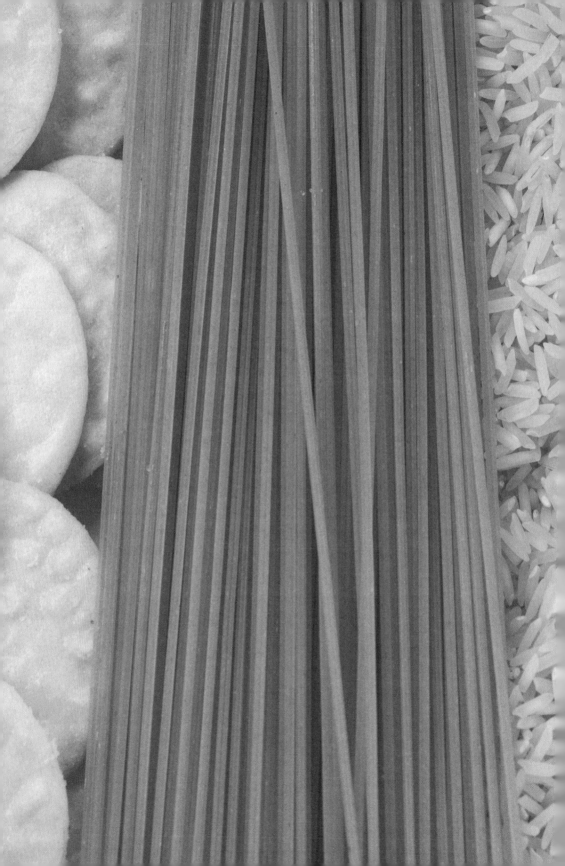

10 common traps

No matter how simple or straightforward LCHF sounds, even the most intelligent people get tripped up by certain aspects. Here are 10 of the most common traps. If you are not making real progress, or feel something is just not right on your journey, come back to these important points.

01 HEARING HALF THE LCHF MESSAGE

No matter how clearly we communicate the message, sometimes people hear only what they want to hear. With LCHF, some people only tend to get half the message – you want to guess which half? That's right, the "eat more fat" half. Taking just half the message and eating more fat without reducing your carbs results in a high-carb, high-fat diet – in other words, the SAD, or Standard American Diet. What a perfect acronym that is! Well, we know exactly how that sort of diet is going, as Americans continue to pave the way for the rest of the world with soaring obesity rates.

I have tried to get the message across in this book and will reiterate it here: HF goes hand in hand with LC – that is, to embrace the LCHF lifestyle, if you increase your fat intake then you MUST reduce your carb intake simultaneously. I urge you to hear both parts of this message. By not doing so, you might end up in a worse state than before you started changing your eating habits at all.

02 MEAT, MEAT, AND MORE MEAT

Whether it's a misinterpreted message of LCHF being a high-protein way of eating, or simply that some people just love their meat, overeating protein is a very common pitfall. The conversion of protein to carbs after a certain threshold is reached is the main reason we need to be mindful of total protein intake. Because I recommend spreading your protein as evenly as possible across all three meals in a day, when it comes to the dinner meal the amount of protein you have left in your allocation is

not that large (about palm size) and often means cutting down to what appears to be a small portion on your plate. This is just a psychological barrier that you need to get over – with enough fat and vegetables on your plate, you should feel satiated without having to eat oversized portions of protein.

03 I SAID MORE FAT

No matter how much you think you will enjoy eating more fat, it does take some time to get your head around it. After years of being told to keep total fat intake low, this adjustment does require a degree of trust. As long as you reduce the carbs simultaneously, you will be okay. More on this in Part 3: Unlocking the real science. Too little fat is likely to leave you hungry, so it's important to increase each meal's fat intake to the point that satiety signals kick in, allowing you to last between main meals without feeling hungry. Not feeling hungry between meals is a good sign that you're eating enough fat. The fact that the LCHF lifestyle doesn't leave you hungry between meals is one of the revolutionary aspects of this approach to eating.

04 SHAKE SOME SALT

A bit like with fat, increasing your salt intake may also seem a bit weird, considering the "low salt" message we've been given for years. But it is very important in the early stages (first week or two) to compensate for the temporary electrolyte imbalance from dropping carbs. Failing to increase your salt intake is likely to make you feel a little "off" at the start. Please take my word for it.

05 CALORIES COUNT

LCHF eating establishes a better interaction of hormones in the body, allowing you to access fat stores for fuel as well as manage your hunger better. But it's still true that if you eat more energy than your body uses, you will gain weight, even on LCHF. It's less likely because you won't feel hungry and it's just harder to overeat fat with a low-carb intake. But in the end, if hunger cues are ignored and you carry on eating, you will gain weight. A good example of this is so-called "healthy" sweet treats. Obviously, replacing the sugar in traditional versions of these sweet treats might make them low carb, but the "treat" still provides extra food (and calories). A treat is a treat, whether it's made from sugar or natural sweetener, and should be limited to infrequent occasions.

06 "GOING NUTS ON NUTS"

I've mentioned this a few times already, but it's so easy to go overboard on nuts that it's worth repeating. While nuts are a great snack, because of the good-quality fat and protein, you must be mindful of your portion sizes. Nuts are very high in total energy (calories) and by "going nuts on nuts," you can easily eat a lot more calories than the body requires. While there is no prescribed limit, as everyone has different needs, as a general rule it would be sensible to have no more than half a cup per day.

07 IT'S OKAY TO ASK

When eating out, people often either forget or don't feel comfortable asking for high-carb items to be removed from their order or replaced. Having these items on your plate can make it tempting to eat them. At that point, all you're relying on is your willpower. It's too easy for "will-power" to turn into "won't-power" – you give in, eat the food, and beat yourself up about it later on. It's far better to nip it in the bud: if the food isn't on your plate, you can't eat it. So next time you're ordering a meal that comes with an obvious "carby" item, just ask for it to be held or replaced with an "LCHF-friendly" option, preferably a vegetable or salad item. You are not being a burden, you're just looking after yourself. You aren't being a pain – they're cooking anyway, and you are paying – you're just being determined to look after your health. Besides, like all things, once you've asked for something to be replaced the first time, it's much easier to ask again.

08 FAKE FOOD

Sugar is hidden in different terminology on food labels. One of the advantages of eating the LCHF way is that deciphering food labels becomes less of an issue because you're eating whole food. However, you also need to be aware of hidden carbs lurking elsewhere. Living in a packaged-food environment means that some speciality items on our shelves (for example, "low-carb" bars) might not be as low in carbs as they appear. Much of this confusion comes from the different labelling laws in different countries, with some manufacturers listing "total carbs" on their labels and others listing "net carbs." "Net carbs" is the carb value counted when the fiber content and the sugar-alcohol (sweetener) content of the product is subtracted from what we know as the total carb count. This happens because these compounds are considered "non-impact" carbs.

Sugar-alcohol sweeteners (called "polyols"), such as sorbitol, xylitol, maltitol, mannitol, and others, are also technically carbs, but we don't completely absorb them. This might sound okay, but in reality these compounds have a glycemic index, causing a rise in blood sugar. And you know what happens when blood sugar rises? Yep, that's right, insulin rises, too – so despite being classed as "non-impact" carbs they have an impact similar to eating carbs.

Glycerine, or glycerol, is also a polyol and is used as a sweetener in packaged foods. While it claims not to have a blood sugar–raising effect, it may have an effect in some insulin-resistant individuals, so some scepticism is warranted here.

Polydextrose, another carbohydrate used as a bulking agent in low-calorie packaged food, claims to have little effect on blood sugar, but is still classed as a carb.

So, if a "low-carb" bar is labeled as containing 5 g of total carbs, but then lists 6 g of fiber, plus 8 g of polydextrose, 7 g of maltitol, and 8 g of glycerine, in reality this adds up to a whopping 34 g of total carbs. So confusing. "Low-carb" bars, due to some clever marketing and labeling, have become a popular snack for many individuals. Now you are informed; best to avoid them.

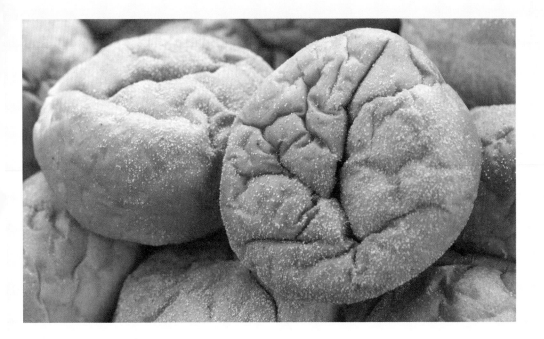

Two take-home messages:
1. Use total carbs for counting purposes.
2. Keep it simple: choose whole foods.

09 GET REAL

Setting unrealistic goals often ends in disappointment, and weight loss is a good example of this. I repeatedly see clients setting unrealistic goal weights – weights they have not seen for many, many years, and sometimes never as an adult. I also see clients setting reasonable weight-loss goals but in an unreasonably short time-frame. Again, un-realistic for long-term sustainability. People often overestimate what they can achieve in the short term and underestimate what they can achieve in the long term. Lots of things change with age and stage and circumstance. Success comes to those who are realistic and patient. Results come easily and instantly for some but might take a little longer for others, especially yo-yo dieters. Patience and perseverance will not only get you there, but will enable you to stay there. Long-term, sustainable weight loss is the ultimate goal. LCHF makes it achievable.

10 "GUT INSTINCT"

The process of changing the way you eat means you have to get to know your body well and actually listen to it. Watch carefully for clues about what to eat, and what not to eat. About when to eat, and when not to eat. Learn the signs: if you don't tolerate a certain food, don't eat it and get the nutrients from a substitute food. You know your body better than anyone else, so be your own science experiment and work out which foods suit and which don't (if any).

If you are unsure, get some help from a well-qualified nutrition professional. Eat when you are hungry, although you may find that your appetite shifts compared with your pre-LCHF days. LCHF eating lends itself to intermittent fasting (IF) for some people. While I don't usually "prescribe" IF to people, if you are not hungry then don't eat. As long as you are getting the required nutrients, and meeting your goals, then missing the occasional meal is not a problem. Listen to your body and follow its needs.

What about alcohol?

Let me begin by saying that alcohol can fit into your *LCHF* lifestyle and overall health. It's just a matter of details.

The idea that alcohol, especially red wine, prevents heart disease might have some truth, but in reality alcohol does cause harm, even in quite small amounts. So the net ratio of harm and benefit in the cardiovascular health context is at best neutral but more likely harmful. Alcohol is a source of empty calories and provides very little else in terms of nutrients. Alcohol can also affect sleep quality, and good sleep is one of the important lifestyle components that goes hand in hand with *LCHF* nutrition on the journey towards optimal living.

Of course, it's not all bad. Alcohol can help people relax and is a social lubricant. For many of us, alcohol can be a pleasurable and important part of life. We enjoy a glass or two of wine with our family or friends. We connect and relax, thereby reducing stress. The positive benefit of this should not be discounted. I would not advocate introducing alcohol if you don't already include it, and I don't advocate stopping it if the small amount you drink genuinely enhances your life. But I do encourage you to aim for at least three or four alcohol-free days each week.

During the initial process of becoming fat adapted, I recommend holding off on alcohol for a week or two, until your body gets settled into its new fat-burning state. You can then gradually reintroduce some alcohol and still achieve your goals. You might also notice that your tolerance for alcohol decreases – so be careful.

There are preferred sources of alcohol, of course, so let's go through them:

Spirits mixed with sugar-containing drinks are by far the highest carb-contributing beverages. Avoid these and replace the sugar-containing beverage with soda water (and freshly squeezed lime or lemon).

Beer contains carbohydrate from left-over maltose derived from the malted grain used in the fermentation process. Low-carb beer has less carbs and is a good occasional option, but don't think it's okay to drink more just because it's low carb. Low-carb beer is not necessarily low in alcohol, and still contains lots of calories from the alcohol itself. The amount of both alcohol and carbohydrate in beer can vary considerably, so do your homework and read the label!

Wine, by definition, is fermented grape juice. It starts off as a sugar-containing fruit, but through the process of adding yeast for fermentation the sugar is converted into ethanol. In sweeter wines, the process of fermentation is stopped before all the sugar turns to ethanol, so they have a higher carb content than drier wines. While drier wines are quite a bit lower in carbs, they still have a fair bit of alcohol and therefore calories.

Liqueurs can be high in carbs and vary considerably between varieties, so avoid regular consumption.

The carb content of popular drinks

Check out the carbohydrate content of a variety of common alcoholic beverages.

Red wine	White wine (sweet)	White wine (dry)	Champagne	Beer	Low-carb beer	Cider	Spirits	Spirit with soft drink	Liqueur
1 glass 100 ml	1 glass 100 ml	1 glass 100 ml	1 glass 100 ml	bottle 340 ml	bottle 340 ml	bottle 330 ml	30 ml	200 ml	30 ml
0 g carbs	2.6 g carbs	0.5 g carbs	1.3 g carbs	10-15 g carbs	3-7 g carbs	8.3 g carbs	0 g carbs	22.9 g carbs	3-17 g carbs

While alcohol in general does not contain a lot of carbohydrate, it still provides energy, contributing 7 calories per gram. Beer, whether it is low carb or standard carb, generally has around 4-5 percent alcohol content, while wines have around 12-15 percent. Cider, which is fermented fruit juice from apples, pears, or other fruits, tends to vary from 4-9 percent alcohol; similarly, spirits also vary widely (15-98 percent).

THE FAT PROFESSOR

I drink some low-carb beer, quite possibly more than I should. I mainly drink low-carb beer when I am at our beach house in Tairua, on the Coromandel in New Zealand - more in summer than in winter. I really enjoy wine, particularly Sauvignon Blanc, the best in the world, from the Marlborough region of New Zealand.

THE WHOLE-FOOD DIETITIAN

I've been officially classified as a "trivial" drinker, on average consuming less than two standard drinks a week. This is true for most weeks of the year, but not for my summer holiday. I spend this at Langs Beach in beautiful Northland, New Zealand. This is where I relax the most, and along with our beachmates we eat, drink, fish, dive, run, bike, play, sing, and relax all day, every day. I enjoy the odd cider, G&T, mojito, and red wine. But my favorite beverage by far is a "BBC" - Big, Buttery Chardonnay.

THE MICHELIN-TRAINED CHEF

Matching wine or beer to a meal can bring the best out of the food - and vice versa. It makes sitting down to eat more of an occasion and creates a good atmosphere for conversation. A crisp glass of white wine with lighter meats and fish, or a full-bodied red with heartier meals, lifts food to the next level. If you go to the effort to prepare something nourishing and tasty, you deserve to relax and enjoy it with a drink of your choosing (possibly not rum and Coke). I believe a single drink with a meal is unlikely to derail your day.

The bottom line: Alcoholic beverages are sources of empty calories; find the balance allowing you to indulge at times while still meeting your goals, whatever they may be.

Your questions answered

In Part 1 of this book, I have tried to provide you with as much practical information about the LCHF lifestyle as possible, but of course the more you learn about it and the more you apply it to your own life, the more questions you are likely to have. Here are my clients' most commonly asked questions.

Q Will I get bored with the meals?

There is a great deal of variety in the foods you can eat with LCHF. With the help of the great recipes and tips *What the Fat?* provides, all that is left to do is some basic and consistent menu planning. Mixing things up a little, rather than eating the same meals day in and day out, is always a good idea. Hence we have provided some variety within each meal category: breakfast, lunch, and dinner. By trying new foods and new combinations of flavors, boredom will not be a problem. Fat makes food taste good, and critically LCHF is easy, varied, and tasty.

Q Is it okay for my children to eat LCHF?

Yes, definitely. LCHF is not necessarily about weight loss, but definitely about health gain, making it suitable for everyone. We recommend this as a whole-family approach. There is no need to cook separate meals for different family members, as LCHF provides all the necessary nutrients for both children and adults to thrive. Remember, this is not a no-carb way of eating, but rather a lower-carb way of eating than mainstream nutritional guidelines traditionally recommend (although they are currently under revision). Carb requirements vary and you can choose to be at the lower or upper end of the spectrum, depending on your goals and how your body reacts.

Q Will I get hungry?

By making use of fat and protein at each meal, the beauty of LCHF is the satiety (feeling of fullness) it provides. People just don't usually feel hungry eating this way. With the increased fat in your meals, and nothing blocking the signals indicating you're full, it's more likely that you will feel less hungry and only require three meals a day, rather

than hankering for snacks between meals. Feeling hungry a couple of hours after a main meal suggests that you consumed insufficient fat (or protein). Depending on your personalized goal, some people do still need snacks, so we have provided some good ideas for you (see page 74).

Q Can I do this if I am vegetarian?

Yes, you definitely can. The level of carbohydrate you might select would depend on the types of animal foods you include in your vegetarian lifestyle, if any. For example, if you eat eggs, fish, or dairy products, then you don't need to get all your protein from vegetable sources such as legumes (which are naturally higher in carbohydrate). If you don't eat any eggs, fish, or dairy and get all your protein from plant-based foods, then you may need to be satisfied with a slightly higher level of carbohydrate so as not to risk compromising protein intake.

Q Can I do this if I am pregnant?

Definitely. However, I would advocate eating at the higher end of the low-carb spectrum and concentrating on the whole-food philosophy. Insulin resistance is a normal occurrence when women become pregnant. Overweight or obese women develop more pronounced insulin resistance during their pregnancy, and they have a higher risk of developing gestational diabetes. For this reason, it is even more important for pregnant women to control the amount of carbohydrate they consume. Remember that carbohydrate, or glucose, is not an essential nutrient, meaning that the body can make enough for its own requirements and that of the fetus, therefore eating the LCHF way will not harm your baby. I don't promote being in ketosis during pregnancy. I don't believe it to be harmful (in the days

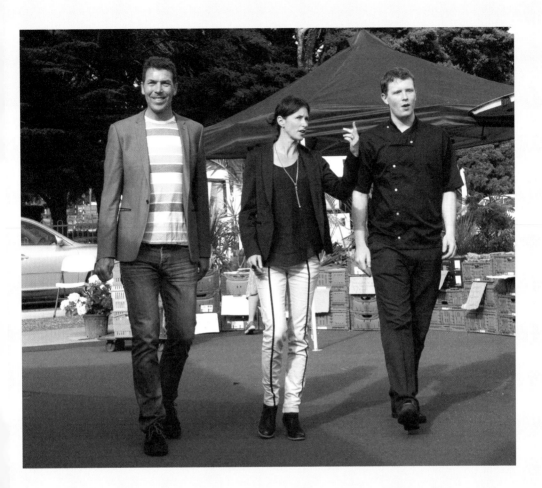

of our ancestors, it would have been common to be in ketosis while pregnant), but because it involves being strict even with vegetables, it might limit necessary nutrients during this important time. I always advise getting nutrients from whole foods rather than from supplementation. Whole foods provide other beneficial nutrients such as fiber and disease-protective natural antioxidants and phytochemicals not available from pills or potions.

Q Can I drink diet soft drinks?

There's no doubt that diet soft drinks are better than full-sugar varieties. However, they contain artificial sweeteners which are still synthetic and not great for the body. If you currently drink full-sugar soft drinks, then I recommend you first replace them with diet soft drinks for a period of time, eventually removing them altogether and replacing them with unsweetened drinks such as water or sparkling water with a squeeze of fresh lemon or lime. Use artificial sweeteners like a heroin addict uses methadone – an aid to get you off the sugar! Ultimately, the aim is to change the "sweet" palate so that you are no longer a slave to sweet cravings.

Q What if I can't eat dairy products?

If you can't tolerate dairy products, then it's important to obtain sufficient protein and calcium from other food sources, such as other types of milk (e.g., almond milk), canned fish (with the bones mashed up) and plenty of vegetables, nuts, and seeds. Whether or not you would need to supplement your diet with a mineral supplement is best determined on an individual basis.

Q Won't I get heart disease if I eat too much red meat?

There is no causative link between eating red meat and getting heart disease. Red meat is an excellent source of protein and micronutrients, particularly iron and zinc. However, I always advise including a range of protein sources each day, including fish, chicken, pork, and eggs, to ensure that a widespread range of nutrients is obtained from all protein foods. This is also a good time to reiterate that LCHF is not about eating a lot of protein, but rather amounts in each meal that your body requires, approximating to palm-sized portions or thereabouts. Do be cautious about processed meats, however. While there is also not a causative link between processed red meat and heart disease, there is some evidence to suggest a relationship between the two, and it is thought that the preservative content could account for this relationship. With this in mind, limit consumption of processed meats.

Q Can you eat too much fat?

Yes, you can, but most people who adopt the LCHF way of eating feel full before they eat too much fat because fat is a satiating nutrient (i.e., it helps keep you full). If you are guided by your satiety and you don't eat for reasons other than providing fuel for the body, you are unlikely to eat too much fat. There are, however, instances when people have strict weight-loss goals where it is important to monitor both total energy intake and carbs. In this case, there is potential to eat too much fat if it is not monitored – fat is calorie-dense and total energy needs can be exceeded if you're not careful. The Easy Diet Diary or a similar app works well to guide you here.

Q Will it be bad for my health?

No. The LCHF lifestyle will be good for your health, both in the short term and in the long term. Eating nutrient-dense whole foods with good-quality fats – and reducing (or eliminating) carbohydrate foods lacking nutritional benefits – promotes optimal health and may even see some existing health issues decrease in severity or be eliminated altogether.

Q How can a diet that eliminates an entire nutrient be healthy?

It is important to realize that LCHF is not about excluding an entire nutrient (i.e., carbs), but rather about choosing the best-quality foods that contain that nutrient. Also, keep in mind that only fat and protein are the essential components that the body cannot produce and that we are reliant on our diet to provide. In contrast, carbohydrate is not an essential nutrient and the body produces enough for our needs. However, we do include some carb foods, for example fruit, vegetables, and dairy products, because these foods also provide other great nutrients such as fiber, vitamins, and minerals.

Q Are lentils and beans protein or carbohydrate?

Lentils and beans are legumes, and typically they provide both of these nutrients as well as a little bit of fat. Each type provides a different profile of nutrients, but, in general, legumes provide two-thirds carbohydrate and one-third protein. They can still be enjoyed as part of a whole-food diet; just be aware that they carry more carbohydrate than other protein sources.

Q How do I know I won't be deficient in nutrients?

Whichever way you decide to eat (high carb, low fat; vegetarian; vegan; or any other way), you need to be mindful about getting sufficient nutrients to prevent nutrient deficiencies. The same applies to LCHF. By including a good amount and a good variety of vegetables, along with a variety of other foods such as dairy, meats (especially organ meats), fruit, nuts, and seeds, you don't need to be concerned about nutrient deficiencies.

Q Can you eat too many eggs?

While there is nothing wrong with eating a few eggs each day, it is a good idea to vary your protein sources over the day to maximize the nutrient profile. For example, if you have eggs for breakfast, then you could have eggs for lunch, too, but it might be a better idea to have a different type of protein. Try salmon, to give you more omega-3 fats, or leftover beef or lamb for a healthy dose of iron.

Q What if I have an emergency sweet craving?

If this craving occurs in the first couple of weeks after adopting the LCHF lifestyle, then I recommend "biting the bullet" and avoiding giving in as much as possible. During this time, your body is going through a withdrawal process from sugar, so naturally it will crave it. The best thing you can do is simply ride it out until the sugar addiction is well and truly gone. If, however, you are well into your LCHF lifestyle but still crave something sweet (this might be around menstruation time for some women), then as long as it is included in your "three-meal" allocation and is considered a "treat" food or occasion, go ahead. However, bear in mind that it is very easy for those carb-addicted feelings and habits to return (in fact, way easier than when you're trying to get rid of them), so just be mindful that this is occasional only. In my experience, clients don't like that sweet-craving feeling – it is often one of their key motivations for going LCHF – so knowing that succumbing will be likely to lead to more cravings can be sufficient motivation to make them turn away from treats and stick to strawberries and cream instead.

Q Is LCHF the same as Paleo?

No, they are not the same, but LCHF and Paleo do share the same whole-food philosophy. Paleo-style eating does not necessarily mean low carb, and while it may end up that way if you follow the whole-food principle, Paleo does not include a restriction on whole-food carbs such as fruit, vegetables, honey, and other natural sugars. LCHF involves a restriction of carbs, even some of the whole-food ones, but this very much depends on what your goal (and level of carb restriction) is. Some Paleo philosophies exclude legumes because they contain anti-nutrients (nutrients that reduce the availability of certain minerals in the body) and can cause gut-related

problems in certain people. Traditional Paleo also excludes dairy products, as these were not consumed in the Paleolithic era (aside from human milk for infants), and due to the belief that milk proteins can promote allergies, inflammation, and autoimmune disease. This viewpoint is not shared by all Paleo advocates. The more modern Paleo movement recommends excluding dairy products only if people are unable to tolerate them. Similarly, the LCHF way of eating includes full-fat dairy products, but also advocates excluding them for those unable to tolerate them.

Q Do I need to exercise?

Regular exercise is extremely important for optimal health. However, the beauty of LCHF is it allows you to control your weight without excessive exercise. Combine some cardio to maintain or increase your overall fitness, and some resistance work to maintain your muscle mass and bone health. But mainly look upon exercise as a regular and enjoyable part of a healthy life.

Q Should I be taking a multivitamin supplement?

No, you won't need to take a multivitamin supplement if you follow the LCHF guidelines properly. Eating a good amount of non-starchy vegetables, preferably at each meal, along with plenty of good, healthy fats and protein provides your body with all the required nutrients. As always, we need to ensure that our busy lifestyles don't get in the way of eating optimal whole foods and therefore risk any nutrient deficiency. LCHF is no exception. Any kind of supplementation needs to be assessed on an individual basis in conjunction with a thorough dietary analysis.

Q Don't I need whole grains for optimal health?

Whole-grain breads and cereal products do provide fiber and vitamins, especially B vitamins, which have been shown to be healthful. This point has never been challenged. However, we can obtain fiber and these same vitamins from other sources of food without the high load of carbohydrate or the anti-nutrients that might reduce the availability of other nutrients in the body. When these manufactured foods are reduced or removed from the diet, it is important to consume a good variety of vegetables, nuts, seeds, and meats (especially organ meats) in their place to obtain the necessary nutrients. Whole foods, which are minimally processed and don't usually come in packages, contain all the nutrients required for optimal health without needing to include whole grains.

Q Can I still do LCHF if I exercise a lot?

Yes, definitely. Many athletes (both recreational and elite) see improvements in health and performance when eating this way. Type, duration, and intensity of exercise must be considered when selecting your level of carb restriction. While carbohydrate (or glucose) is often used for fuel during exercise, fat is also an excellent (if not better) fuel source for exercise. Even the leanest of us have a lot more fat stores that can be used for fuel than the limited carbohydrates stored in our muscles. Using fat as your primary fuel source during exercise is the best scenario, only drawing on carbohydrate to fuel high-intensity bursts. This will occur if you are a fat-burner or are "fat adapted," as discussed on page 42.

Q Is LCHF a fad diet?

We've discussed this before, but it's worth re-iterating. LCHF is definitely not a fad diet; it is a lifestyle choice. I do not endorse fad diets, or any diets for that matter: embarking on a diet implies that you will stop it at some point and revert to your previous way of eating. I don't advocate doing this, as any improvements in health and well-being that you experience on LCHF are likely to disappear if you revert to old eating habits.

Q Isn't this just the Atkins diet?

True, LCHF has similarities to the Atkins diet. However, Atkins has a greater focus on protein and less of a focus on vegetables and good-quality fats. It also includes the promotion of packaged Atkins-branded food items such as bars and shakes. In contrast, LCHF advocates whole food (i.e., unpackaged foods), focuses particularly on vegetables, and encourages a moderate protein intake.

Q Is it okay to use alternative sweeteners?

Artificial sweeteners are just that . . . artificial, and one of the main concepts of the LCHF lifestyle is to eat food that aligns with how nature intended us to eat. So, while many studies show that artificial sweeteners are not harmful, it is my preference not to use them. Firstly, if you want that sweet taste you could use a natural sweetener such as stevia (which comes from a plant). Secondly, and probably most importantly, the idea of LCHF eating is to alter your "sweet" palate so you don't end up craving sweet things all the time. Consuming sweet foods, regardless of whether they contain sugar, prolongs the addiction to sugar. Therefore, any sweet item is best viewed as an infrequent treat.

Q Can I get enough fiber on LCHF?

Yes. Done properly, you can get more beneficial fiber (i.e., soluble fiber) eating the LCHF way. This means eating a good amount of vegetables (mainly those non-starchy vegetables listed on page 66), and some fruit and nuts. These foods provide all the fiber you need.

Done well, LCHF will benefit the whole family.

Proof LCHF helps Type 1 Diabetes

TRISH BRADBURY, 55, UNIVERSITY LECTURER

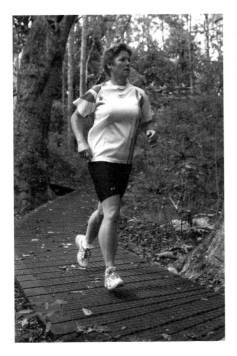

When I was diagnosed with diabetes 25 years ago, it was a bit of a shock as I ate well and was pretty fit. I didn't know much about diabetes, but my attitude was to just get on with things and lead a normal life. I thought, "Well, I just have to keep eating healthily and stay fit for the rest of my life." In recent years, I have moved along with technology and switched to an insulin pump. I track my blood sugar and program the pump to deliver the required insulin (which I can't produce myself – that's what a Type 1 diabetic is) to maintain my blood sugar at between 6 and 6.4 mmol/L.

Part of the problem with being a Type 1 diabetic is you get "hypos," which happen when you fail to match your carb intake and insulin properly; that is, you eat too few carbs and have more insulin in your body than you need. This results in low blood sugar, which can have severe consequences if you're not careful, as hypos can lead to blacking out. One time, I was out swimming by myself in the ocean, training for a half-ironman, when I had a hypo. Luckily, I was close to shore and was rescued by someone walking on the beach. I tried to get back in the water, but he pulled me out again and called the paramedics. I don't want to think about what could have happened if he had not been there.

The big advantage I have noticed from LCHF is that even if my blood sugar goes low, the effect isn't too severe. I am much more "hypo-proof" on LCHF. Other advantages include:

- I have effortlessly dropped several pounds
- My HbA1c has dropped from 8.8 percent to 6.2 percent
- My insulin use is down by 30 percent (from 30 units per day to 21)
- My blood cholesterol results are awesome; they were awesome before, but importantly they are still awesome, even though I eat loads of fat
- I have heaps of energy and feel great.

One thing that helped along the way is that this became a social thing with my friends. We were all giving it a go. So going LCHF was pretty cool and we are all into working out how many carbs were in different foods and what some yummy foods to eat are. It's been fun and it's really cool that LCHF suits my style of eating, my health, and my diabetes. The main barrier for me was getting information. I needed this book!

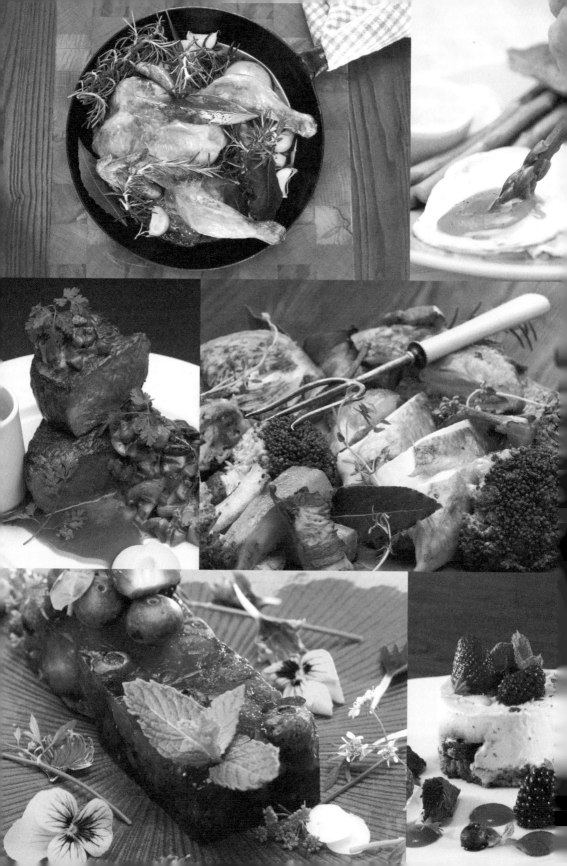

Part 2
Your new
LCHF menu

Hi, it's me, Craig.

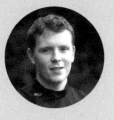

The following recipes are straightforward and user-friendly, since a recipe is just words on a page unless someone actually COOKS it! Each recipe has its own suggested number of servings. If you are cooking for others, simply multiply the recipe for the number you want. In my recipes, I have listed the ingredients in both grams and milliliters and the more user-friendly cups and tablespoons to enable the recipes to be easily and universally replicated.

I have to confess that as a chef I have a pet dislike for the cup/tablespoon system, as it relies much more on approximate weights based on volume (in the restaurant, we even weigh liquids in grams, for accuracy, instead of using milliliters). Be aware that a standard measuring cup is probably a different size from the mug in your cupboard. For liquid volumes, we have used the metric standards: 1 cup is equal to 250 ml, 1 tsp (teaspoon) is equal to 5 ml, 1 Tbsp (tablespoon) is equal to 15 ml, etc. For cuts of meat or fish, ask your butcher or fishmonger for the weight you require, or use supermarket labels as a guide.

The recipes in each section progress from easy, everyday meals to more challenging ones for entertaining or when you have time to put some real effort in. The dishes in the book are designed to be flexible – feel free to add or omit ingredients according to your preference. As you grow familiar with the basic recipes, you will build up your own repertoire of skills to take your cooking and eating to another level. LCHF is a lifestyle and a cuisine in its own right; that's why it's important to embrace cooking to fully understand that the most nutritious meals you will eat are likely to be the ones you cook for yourself.

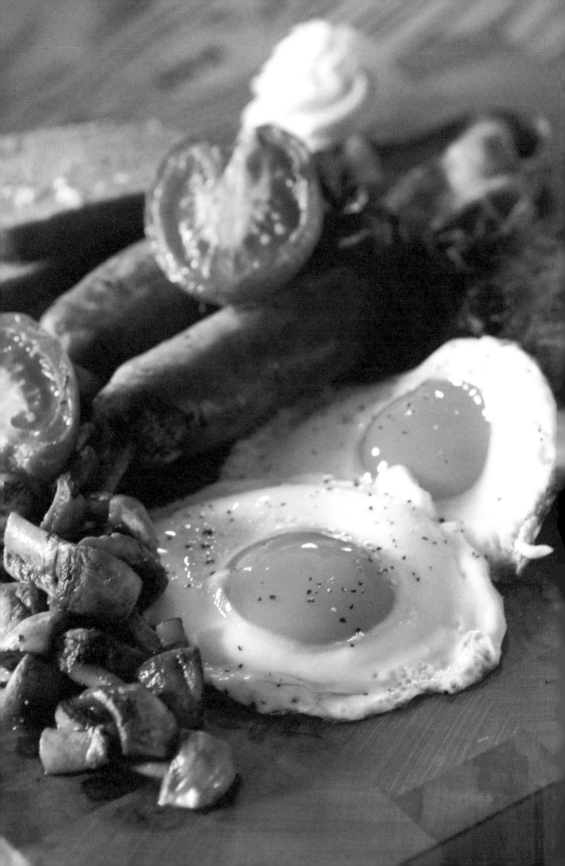

Breakfast

LCHF allows for flexibility at breakfast. Some people are more hungry in the morning and we have recipes that will produce delicious, substantial meals; but for people who like to start light, you can still begin your day in the right way. Have a smoothie or grab a crustless quiche; even a simple coffee with cream will represent what some people start the day off with in their LCHF life.

Boiled eggs

Quick, convenient and amazing, eggs are so versatile. Added to make any meal heartier, or forming a meal on their own, there are some trade secrets to cooking them well – so here's a refresher course in the art of the egg.

Serves	1
Prep time	1 minute
Cooking time	3–10 minutes
Carb count	0.5 g (2 eggs)

EQUIPMENT
Pot, timer, slotted spoon, bowl of cold water

INGREDIENTS
2 eggs

METHOD
Put the eggs in a pot and add an inch of water to cover. Put the pot on the highest heat until it comes to a boil. Remove from the heat and start the timer – leaving the egg in the hot water off the heat gives a more consistent result. How the egg is cooked is to your own preference: 10 minutes produces a hard-boiled egg (without that green-line effect); 2 minutes produces a very soft-boiled egg; I find 3–4 minutes is perfect. Boiled eggs can be cooled in cold water to eat cold or have later. They store well in the fridge, making a quick snack or a tasty component in something like a Caesar salad.

Poached eggs

Every hotel in the world pre-poaches eggs; it is the only way to serve hundreds of people breakfast. Pre-poaching is useful at home, too, when you are cooking for a few people.

Serves	1
Prep time	1 minute
Cooking time	5 minutes
Carb count	0.5 g (2 eggs)

EQUIPMENT
Pot, whisk, timer, slotted spoon, bowl of cold water (if pre-poaching)

INGREDIENTS
1 liter (1 quart) water
50 ml (just under ¼ cup) vinegar
2 eggs

METHOD
Put the water in the pot and bring to a boil. Add the vinegar and reduce the heat until the water no longer boils. Create a current in the pot by moving the whisk around the inside a couple of times – this helps shape the egg and prevents it from sinking and flattening on the bottom. Crack 1 egg into the water and stir the water a couple more times with the slotted spoon to help the current regain a bit of speed; this allows the next egg to get the same nice shape as the first. Try to add the remainder of the eggs you require in less than 30 seconds, to avoid overcooking the first egg. Start the timer, and after 2 minutes check if the eggs are ready – they should feel soft, but the outside should be firm enough that you can lift them out of the water with the slotted spoon without breaking them.

To pre-poach the eggs, cook them in batches and cool them quickly in the bowl of cold water. Cooked eggs will keep very well for up to 3 days. Reheating the eggs takes about 1 minute in the poaching water brought back up to 212°F.

Scrambled eggs

Many fine restaurants test new chefs' skills by challenging them to demonstrate a couple of basic egg techniques – they very quickly illustrate whether a chef can actually "cook"!

Serves   1
Prep time   2 minutes
Cooking time   5 minutes
Carb count   0.6 g (2 eggs)

EQUIPMENT
Nonstick pot, bowl, whisk, spatula

INGREDIENTS
20 g (1½ Tbsp) butter
2 eggs
salt and pepper to taste

METHOD
Melt the butter in the pot and remove from the heat. Whisk the eggs in the bowl and pour into the pot. Return the pot to the heat and slowly whisk. I was taught that the egg "curds" ought to be as small as possible and that the eggs should be cooked only to the point where they are creamy and soft ("baveuse"). To do this you have to let the heat in the pot finish the cooking, so once they are beginning to set, remove the pot from the heat and continue to whisk. Add the seasoning and return the pot to the heat only if you're sure they need more cooking. There are a million things you can add to scrambled eggs; I love to add a handful of spinach and diced tomatoes at the end to make them more interesting.

Omelette

The traditional method of cooking an omelette is quite a skillful technique – encasing a scrambled egg center within a skin of cooked egg. The alternative method here does mean that you need an oven or broiler to finish the cooking, but it is a lot simpler!

Serves   1
Prep time   5 minutes
Cooking time   6–8 minutes
Carb count   4.6 g

EQUIPMENT
Nonstick ovenproof frying pan, whisk, bowl, spatula

INGREDIENTS
20 g (1½ Tbsp) butter
2 eggs
15 g (2 Tbsp) grated cheese, your choice
    (mozzarella and cheddar work well)
100 g (1 small) tomato, diced
15 g (½ cup) baby spinach
50 g (⅓ cup) diced bell pepper

METHOD
Preheat the oven to 350°F. Melt the butter in the frying pan over medium heat. Whisk the eggs in the bowl and add them to the pan. As the underneath cooks, gently push the sides in to allow the raw egg mixture to pour into the space. When there is no more runny egg but the top of the omelette is still moist, add the fillings on top of the eggs and put the pan into the oven for 3 minutes. The eggs should be cooked through; if not, check again at 1-minute intervals. Fold the omelette if you like, or just slide it onto a plate.

Crustless quiche muffins

These keep well in the fridge for at least three days and are the ideal go-to when you need to grab something on the run. Accompany with a small salad and a handful of nuts for a nourishing small breakfast.

Makes	6 large or 12 small muffins
Prep time	15 minutes
Cooking time	12 minutes
Carb count	3 g per serving

EQUIPMENT

Nonstick muffin pan (greased), baking sheet (to go under muffin pan if flimsy), chopping board, knife, frying pan, bowl, whisk

INGREDIENTS

30 g (2 Tbsp) butter
50 g (½ cup) diced onion
50 g (⅔ cup) diced mushrooms
1-2 slices bacon, diced (optional)
5 g (1 tsp) chopped herbs (any you have
   on hand)
20 g (1 generous Tbsp) chopped sun-dried
   tomatoes
5 g (2 tsp) toasted pine nuts (allow 3 minutes in
   oven at 350°F to toast)
salt and pepper to taste
6 eggs
125 ml (½ cup) cream
50 g (1½ cups) arugula (or ¾ cup kale works, too)
50-75 g (1½-2½ oz) cheese, grated (6-10 Tbsp)
   (strong cheddar or a crumbly feta)

METHOD

Preheat the oven to 325°F. Melt the butter in the frying pan over medium heat and sweat the onions, mushrooms, and bacon (if using) over medium heat for 3-5 minutes, until they have lost their moisture and are beginning to caramelize. Take off the heat and add in the herbs, sun-dried tomatoes, toasted pine nuts, and seasoning. Crack the eggs into the bowl and whisk until completely combined. Whisk in the cream and then season again. Evenly divide the fried mixture among the muffin cup slots, add some arugula and a little cheese (reserve some cheese for on top), and fill with the egg mixture until a little below the top of the muffin cups. Top with the remaining cheese and bake in the oven until just set. Depending on the depth of your muffin pan, this can take from 8-15 minutes.

These crustless quiches can be served warm straight away, or kept and served cold straight from the fridge, warmed in the oven for 5 minutes, or warmed for 20 seconds in the microwave if you're in a hurry. Add any alterations you like - smoked salmon or other smoked fish are excellent in these, especially with a spoonful of horseradish in the egg mix.

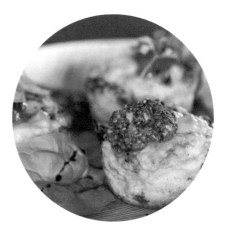

Continental breakfast

This quick, satisfying breakfast can be made effortless by having a batch of cooked vegetables on hand that you might have used for the previous day's dinner or lunch. Cured meats keep really well and a little goes a long way.

Serves	1
Prep time	8 minutes
Cooking time	4-10 minutes
Carb count	16.1 g

EQUIPMENT

Chopping board, knife, ovenproof dish, pot of water, timer

INGREDIENTS

1 slice Low-Carb Bread (page 156)
30 g (½ small) roasted carrot
30 g (small piece) roasted parsnip
1 egg
40 g (3-4 slices) cured meats (selection of ham, salami, prosciutto, speck, bresaola, pepperoni, chorizo, pancetta, etc.)
20 g (⅔ cup) spinach
6-7 olives
½ avocado
15 g (2 Tbsp) almonds
20 g (½ oz) cheese (whatever is your favorite; cheddar or brie work well)
5 g (1 tsp) butter

METHOD

Preheat the oven to 350°F. Place the slice of low-carb bread in the ovenproof dish. Add the carrot and parsnip (or whatever leftover vegetable you have) to the dish next to the bread, and put it in the oven for 5 minutes to warm. Boil or poach (page 96) the egg. Arrange the cured meats, spinach, olives, avocado, almonds, and cheese on the plate, then add the warm vegetables and the egg. Serve with the warm bread, buttered.

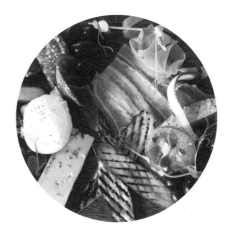

Grain-free granola with yogurt & berries

Grain-free granola is a versatile ingredient that can be used as a topping for desserts or simply enjoyed with yogurt and berries, as in this recipe. Using a packet of mixed nuts or grabbing small amounts from the bulk-bin section of the supermarket means you won't have to buy too many at once. Nuts are pricey, but buying in bulk reduces the price of them in the long run. Remember to buy raw nuts wherever possible, as some pre-roasted ones come in oils we want to avoid.

Makes	about 20 servings
Prep time	10 minutes
Cooking time	10 minutes
Carb count	14.8 g per serving

EQUIPMENT

Ovenproof dish, 2 large plates, food processor or mortar and pestle, large mixing bowl, wooden spoon, storage jar

INGREDIENTS

200 g (1½ cups) almonds
200 g (1½ cups) hazelnuts
200 g (1¾ cups) pecans
200 g (1¾ cups) walnuts
200 g (1½ cups) macadamia nuts
125 g (¾ cup) flaxseed
200 g (1½ cups) pumpkin seeds/pepitas
200 g (1½ cups) sunflower seeds
200 g (2½ cups) coconut flakes (shredded/ desiccated works fine, too)
50 g (6 Tbsp) grated dark chocolate (85% cocoa or higher)
optional pinch of spices: cinnamon, nutmeg, cardamom

TO SERVE, PER PERSON

80 g (⅓ cup) full-fat, unsweetened plain yogurt
50 g (⅓–½ cup) fresh or frozen berries

METHOD

Preheat the oven to 350°F. Toast the nuts in the ovenproof dish for 5 minutes, stir, and then toast for 2–3 minutes longer to cook evenly. Transfer the nuts to the large plates to cool for 10 minutes. Put the cooled nuts into the food processor and pulse in 1-second bursts until they are chopped to the size you like. Pour the nuts into the bowl and stir in the seeds, coconut, chocolate, and the spices, if using. Mix well and then transfer to the storage jar to keep fresh. This granola will stay fresh for up to 1 month in a cool, dark place, so scale up the recipe if you want more. To serve, spoon the yogurt and berries into a bowl and top with the granola.

TIP

While you have the oven on, it's a good idea to make extra toasted nuts for other recipes. They keep for up to 2 weeks in an airtight container. Take care not to burn softer nuts like cashews – underdone is better than over!

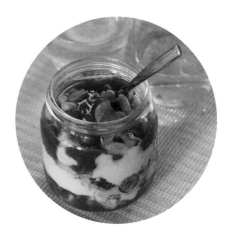

Chia seed porridge with yogurt & berries

Serves   1
Prep time   5 minutes
Standing time at least 30 minutes
Carb count   14.8 g

EQUIPMENT
Serving bowl, whisk or fork, chopping board, knife, measuring cup

INGREDIENTS
125 ml (½ cup) almond milk or coconut milk
30 g (3 Tbsp) chia seeds
stevia (or xylitol) to taste
40 g (2½ Tbsp) full-fat, unsweetened plain yogurt
2 g (1 tsp) cocoa powder
15 g (2 Tbsp) mixed nuts
25 g (¼ cup) fresh (or frozen) berries

METHOD
Combine the milk, chia seeds, and stevia in the bowl. Mix very well with the whisk or fork for 20 seconds, then let the mixture stand for 10 minutes and whisk again. Cover and place the bowl in the fridge for at least 30 minutes. A longer time (e.g., overnight) is better if you want a thicker porridge; if it comes out too thick, you can stir in a little more liquid.

Top the thickened porridge with the plain yogurt and dust with cocoa. Top this off with the nuts and berries. If you like, add a teaspoon of store-bought almond butter.

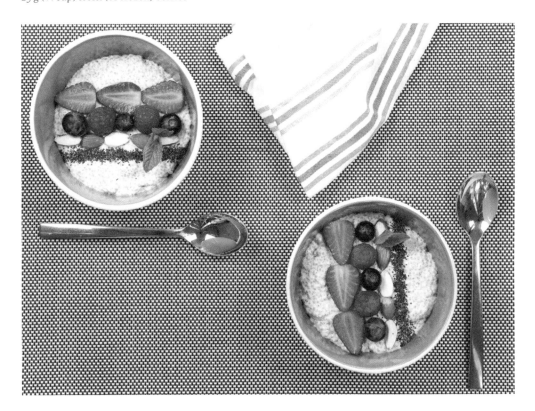

Green power smoothie

*This is an excellent way to ensure you are eating
your phytonutrient-dense greens. The combination
and ratios of ingredients in this recipe are a suggestion
only – if you prefer a different green leaf (or if it's
more seasonal), swap it in.*

Serves	2
Prep time	10 minutes
Carb count	11 g per serving

EQUIPMENT
Chopping board, knife, hand blender or
stand blender

INGREDIENTS
50 g (1½ cups) spinach
50 g (¾ cup) kale
5 g (1 tsp) crushed ginger
½ avocado
½ small cucumber
1 apple, core removed
1 clove garlic, peeled
10 g (2 Tbsp) pumpkin seeds/pepitas
10 g (3 Tbsp) sunflower seeds
water, depending on consistency

METHOD
Blend all the ingredients together, adding water if
necessary to achieve a good consistency.

Very berry smoothie

*Antioxidant-rich berries are naturally low in carbs
and are delicious and versatile. Use fresh berries when
in season and frozen mixed berries during the rest of
the year. Frozen berries are great, as they add a nice
cold edge to the drink and change the texture.*

Serves	1
Prep time	8 minutes
Carb count	12.2 g

EQUIPMENT
Hand blender or stand blender

INGREDIENTS
30 g (4 medium) strawberries
30 g (¼ cup) blueberries
30 g (¼ cup) raspberries
125 ml (½ cup) coconut milk
50 ml (just under ¼ cup) water
10 g (2 Tbsp) pumpkin seeds/pepitas
10 g (3 Tbsp) sunflower seeds

METHOD
Remove the stems from the strawberries if they
are fresh. Blend all the ingredients together
until smooth.

Hazelnut & chocolate iced mocha

Okay. Summertime. Weekend. Friends around for brunch. Something fun and easy to start the day. Serve alongside some berries and cream for a decadent, guilt-free breakfast. Add a pre-prepared sharing side of the Continental Breakfast (page 99) or Chia Seed Porridge (page 101) and feed a gaggle of friends without being distracted by cooking, or scale down the recipe and treat yourself if you're on your own.

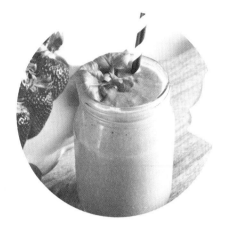

Serves	3-4
Prep time	10 minutes
Carb count	7.4 g per serving

EQUIPMENT

Hand blender or stand blender, measuring cup

INGREDIENTS

200 ml (¾ cup) cream (plus extra for whipping, optional)

80 g (3 oz) dark chocolate (85% cocoa or higher)

40 g (5 Tbsp) toasted hazelnuts (see page 100 for instructions)

625 ml (2⅔ cups) cold coffee (made however you usually make it)

7-8 ice cubes

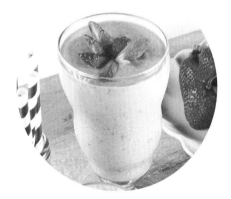

METHOD

Blend the cream, chocolate, and hazelnuts for 10 seconds or so. After the mixture is sufficiently blended, pour in the coffee and blend for a second or two to incorporate the coffee. Serve in a tall glass with ice. Alternatively, add the ice cubes at the beginning so that they get blended in.

If you want to garnish with a topping of whipped cream, save yourself the washing up by whipping it in the unwashed blender.

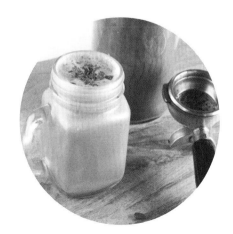

Almond pancakes with bacon & mascarpone

These pancakes are incredibly popular in the restaurant. We've been caught needing to make a fresh mix a couple of times during service, thinking, "Surely we have enough now!" The mix lasts well and improves with time, lasting up to three or four days if kept covered in the fridge.

Serves	2–3
Prep time	10 minutes
Cooking time	10 minutes
Carb count	4.8 g per serving

EQUIPMENT

Mixing bowl, whisk, frying pan, fish slice, large plate, clean dish cloth

INGREDIENTS

10 g (2 tsp) olive oil, coconut oil, or clarified butter

Pancake batter

100 g (1 cup) almond meal
1 egg
60 ml (¼ cup) water
15 g (1 Tbsp) melted butter
a few drops stevia (or xylitol)
small pinch salt

Topping (per person)

3 slices bacon
15 g (1 Tbsp) mascarpone
6–7 berries for garnish
berry purée to serve (optional; see page 162)

METHOD

Mix all the pancake batter ingredients well with the whisk. Allow to rest for 10 minutes. Heat the frying pan over medium heat and add the oil or clarified butter. Spoon dollops of the pancake mixture into the pan. The pancakes should take about 1 minute to color on the first side – any quicker, and the pan is too hot. Turn the pancakes and allow to cook for 1 minute longer. Transfer the pancakes to the plate and cover with the clean dishcloth (the cloth absorbs the steam, so it doesn't make them soggy - great tip from my mum!). Panfry the bacon over medium heat until slightly golden. Arrange the pancakes on the plate with the bacon and mascarpone, and serve with berries on top. Drizzle with berry purée if desired.

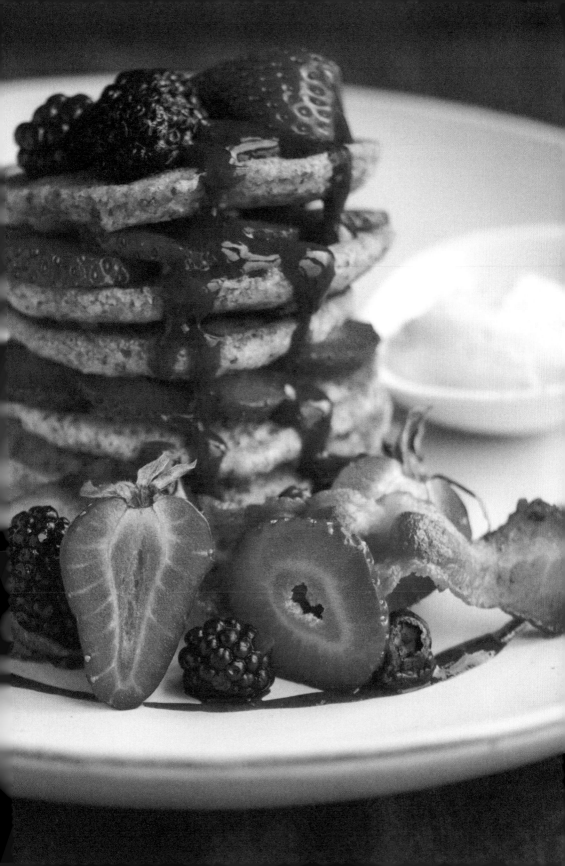

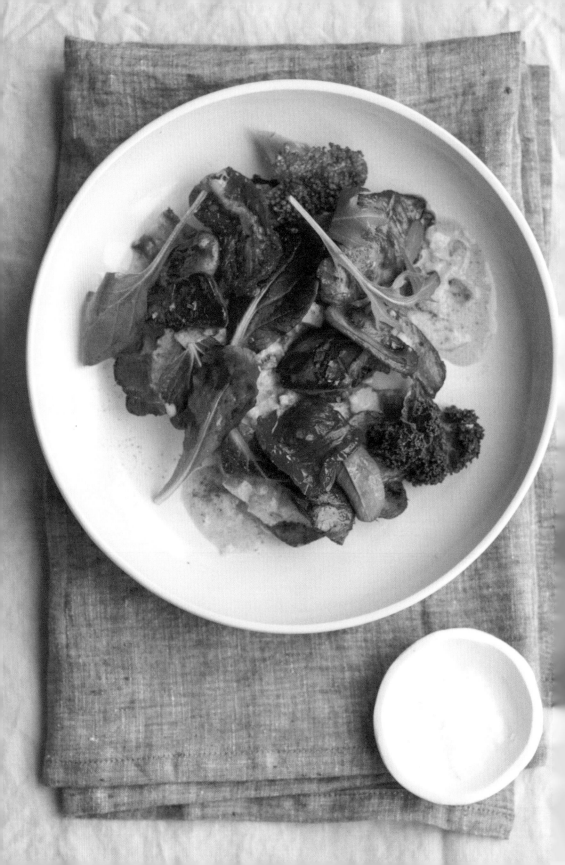

Smoky mushrooms & sun-dried tomatoes with chicken livers on toast

Livers are a nutritional powerhouse. This recipe incorporates livers in a quick meal that is satisfying and nourishing.

Serves	1
Prep time	10 minutes
Cooking time	12 minutes
Carb count	8.2 g

EQUIPMENT

Frying pan, chopping board, knife, bowl, toaster

INGREDIENTS

25 g (¼ small) onion

50 g (10-12) button or cremini mushrooms, sliced

2 slices prosciutto or pancetta (or bacon), chopped or whole

10 g (2 tsp) butter

10 ml (2 tsp) coconut oil, clarified butter, or olive oil, for cooking

80 g (3 oz) chicken livers

30 ml (2 Tbsp) cream

50 g (1½ cups) spinach or blanched broccoli (⅓ cup), plus extra to garnish

5 g (1 tsp) Pesto (page 131)

10 g (2 tsp) chopped sun-dried tomatoes

2 slices Low-Carb Bread (page 156, loaf pan variation)

METHOD

Fry the onion, mushrooms, and prosciutto or pancetta in the butter over medium heat until the water content has evaporated and the ingredients are beginning to caramelize. Remove the mix from the pan, clean the pan, and then reheat it until hot. Add the cooking oil, and when almost smoking-hot add the livers. When the livers are browned on one side, turn them and return the onion, mushrooms, and prosciutto or pancetta to the pan. Pour in the cream and add the spinach or blanched broccoli and the pesto. Add the sun-dried tomatoes.

Toast the slices of bread in the toaster and serve with the smoky mushroom mixture on top. Garnish with extra greens.

Cooked breakfast (big breakfast)

LCHF redeems the time-honored glutton's choice. With the inclusion of vegetable sides, it is now back on the menu as a nourishing way to start the day.

Serves 2
Prep time 15 minutes
Cooking time 20 minutes
Carb count 10.8 g (per serving)

EQUIPMENT

Ovenproof dish, grater, frying pan, mixing bowl, chopping board, knife, spoon, spatula

INGREDIENTS

200 g (7–8 oz; 2) your favorite sausages
4 slices bacon (optional)

Rösti

50 g (½ small) onion
15 g (1 Tbsp) butter
50 g (1 small) zucchini
50 g (½ small) Italian or Asian eggplant
1 egg, beaten
15 g (2 Tbsp) grated Parmesan (optional)

2 tomatoes, halved
60 g (¼ cup) butter, for cooking
100 g (4 oz; 15–20) button mushrooms
2 eggs
100 g (generous 3 cups) spinach
salt and pepper to taste

METHOD

Preheat the oven to 350°F. Place the sausages, and bacon if using, in the preheated oven, in an ovenproof dish large enough to hold all the other items.

To make the rösti, grate the onion and sweat with the butter in the frying pan over medium heat. Grate the zucchini and eggplant into the bowl. Squeeze some water out of the grated vegetables and discard. Add the hot onions to the rest of the vegetables and leave to stand for 5 minutes, until cool enough to add the beaten egg and the Parmesan, if using. Mix well, season, and leave to rest for 5 minutes.

After 10–12 minutes, the sausages will be nearly cooked. Place the tomato halves face down in the ovenproof dish beside the sausages for 5 minutes to cook through; add a little butter to the dish if necessary. Wipe out the frying pan and melt some more butter over medium heat. Using the spoon, scoop some rösti mix into the pan and fry both sides until they begin to color. Transfer the cooked rösti to the ovenproof dish to keep warm. Sauté the mushrooms in a little butter until beginning to color, then season. Fry the eggs in a little more butter, then season. Wilt the spinach in a touch of butter for only about 30 seconds, retaining some life in the spinach. Remove the ovenproof dish from the oven and arrange the items on a plate. Add a slice of Low-Carb Bread (page 156) per person if you wish.

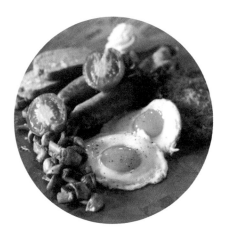

Eggs benedict

I was once told not to put eggs benedict on a breakfast menu at a French restaurant in Auckland because it was "too Kiwi." Be that as it may, this French classic is easily made LCHF by upgrading the bread part of the recipe with a choice of alternatives to boring old English muffins and the like.

Serves 4-5
Prep time 15 minutes
Cooking time 20 minutes
Carb count 3.5 g per serving

EQUIPMENT
Bowl of cold water, empty pot, jug, mixing bowl, whisk, pot of simmering water, frying pan, timer, slotted spoon

INGREDIENTS
2 poached eggs (see page 96 for instructions)

**Hollandaise sauce
(serves 4-5 based on 2-3 Tbsp per serving)**
250 g (1 cup) butter
2 egg yolks
5 ml (1 tsp) white wine vinegar or cider vinegar
15 ml (1 Tbsp) water
salt and pepper to taste
5 g (small pinch) chopped chives (optional)

2 slices Low-Carb Bread (page 156), or Rösti (page 108)
8-10 slices (2 per person) bacon
15 g (1 Tbsp) butter
100 g (generous 3 cups) spinach

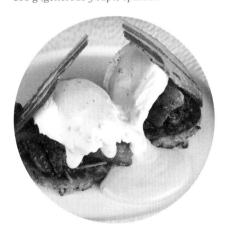

METHOD
Poach the eggs (see page 96) and reserve them in the bowl of cold water.

To make the hollandaise, melt the butter in the empty pot. Pour the melted butter into the jug and allow to stand for 5 minutes while the oil portion of the butter rises to the top; it is this oil portion that is used to make the hollandaise sauce. Add the egg yolks, vinegar, and water to the mixing bowl. Begin whisking the mixture, then place the bowl on top of the pot of simmering water. The heat from the pot will slowly increase the temperature of the yolk mixture and will help to pasteurize the eggs, as well as establishing the thick "sabayon" that is the base for making the hollandaise.

If you are serving your eggs benedict with reheated rösti, Preheat the oven to 325°F.

Continue to whisk the egg yolk mixture until it has thickened and feels warm-to-hot to the touch. Remove the bowl from the heat and place the bowl over the empty pot for stability. Begin whisking in the melted butter, using only the oily top portion, pouring it from the jug in a slow, steady stream; this will take about 2 minutes. Once the hollandaise is made, season with salt and pepper and add the chives, if using.

Toast the low-carb bread, or reheat the rösti in the oven, and place on the plate. Panfry the bacon and place on the side of the plate. To the same pan, add the butter and the spinach. Toss together until wilted, season, and sit the spinach on top of the toast or rösti. Reheat the eggs in the pot of boiling water for 60 seconds, then drain well on paper towels, season, and place on top of the spinach. Sit the bacon on top of the eggs and sauce the benedict as generously as you like.

Huevos rancheros

Mexican ranchers' eggs. Spicy and satisfying, a great start to the day and so easy to put together.

Serves	3-4
Prep time	15 minutes
Cooking time	2 hours (15 minutes if you have your ground meat ready)
Carb count	6.1 g per serving

EQUIPMENT

Pot with lid, chopping board, knife; if boiling or poaching eggs: pot of boiling water, whisk, timer and slotted spoon; if scrambling eggs: nonstick frying pan

INGREDIENTS

500 g (1 lb) ground meat (beef, pork, lamb, or chicken all work well)
1 onion, diced
1 carrot, diced
1 clove garlic, crushed
one 14.5-oz can tomatoes
3 g (½ tsp) tomato paste
5 g (1 tsp) chili powder (or more if you like it hot)
30 g (2 Tbsp) Tomato Salsa (page 133)
30 g (2 Tbsp) Guacamole (page 133)
2 thin slices Low-Carb Bread (page 156), cut into triangles
3-4 eggs (1 per person)
30 g (2 Tbsp) sour cream
20 g (½ oz) cheddar cheese, grated (2 Tbsp)

METHOD

Preheat the oven to 325°F. Start by making the chili. Cook the ground meat in the pot over medium heat, allowing the fat to render out. Add the onion, carrot, and garlic. Cook the vegetables and meat mix for 5-8 minutes, until it has begun to brown and the vegetables are releasing their water. Add in the canned tomatoes, the tomato paste, and the chili powder (adding extra if you like it spicy), cover with the lid, and allow to cook for 1-2 hours. The chili can be made well in advance - it improves over the course of a day or two. It also freezes well, and provided you have a large pot, is easy to make in a big batch.

If you haven't made them already, make the tomato salsa and guacamole. Toast the low-carb bread triangles in the oven. Cook the eggs as you like, from poached (page 96) to scrambled (page 97) to fried. Place the chili in serving bowls and top with the salsa, guacamole, sour cream, cheese, and eggs, scattering the toasted triangles around the bowl.

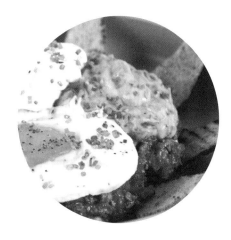

Fish kedgeree

A breakfast dish that's tasty at any time of the day, and a great way to use up food items you have on hand.

Serves	1
Prep time	5 minutes
Cooking time	15 minutes
Carb count	3.5 g

EQUIPMENT

Small pot with a lid, chopping boards, knives, pot of boiling water

INGREDIENTS

60 ml (¼ cup) cream

60 ml (¼ cup) water

150 g (5 oz) white fish fillet (sole, cod, or similar)

salt and pepper to taste

1 poached egg (see page 96 for instructions)

50 g (½ cup) Cauliflower Pilau (page 154)

75 g (½ cup) cooked green vegetables (broccoli, asparagus, green beans)

pinch of turmeric

METHOD

Put the cream, water, and fish in the small pot. Bring to a boil and season. Place the lid on, take off the heat, and leave to gently cook through for 5 minutes. Meanwhile, poach the egg (see page 96) and drain. Remove the cooked fish from the pot and set aside. Add the cauliflower pilau to the creamy liquid in the pot and put back on high heat for 1 minute. Add in the cooked vegetables to reheat along with the pilau. Serve the pilau and vegetables with the fish, topped with the poached egg and seasoned again with salt and pepper, plus a pinch of turmeric for flavoring.

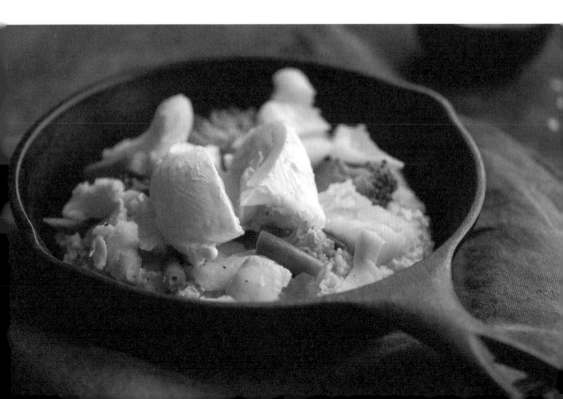

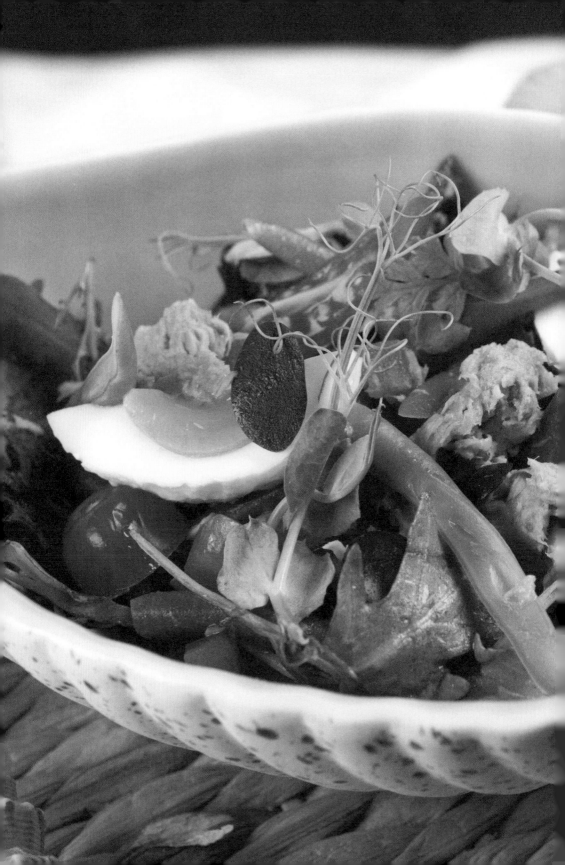

Lunch

Lunch is often the meal that causes problems when you're attempting to change your eating habits. If you've had a particularly busy time, it can be difficult to stay organized enough to feed yourself well on the run. These recipes are designed to show you how to use food you might have around. By pairing it with some fresh salads, vegetables, and dressings, you can have a ton of options that allow you to eat well without having to resort to the best the cafés have to offer.

Soup kitchen

Soup is surprisingly quick and easy to make. Grab some from the fridge or freezer, and in 10 minutes you have a satisfying meal. Armed with some reliable containers, it's easy to take to work and reheat, or take in a Thermos flask and top up your cup with soup.

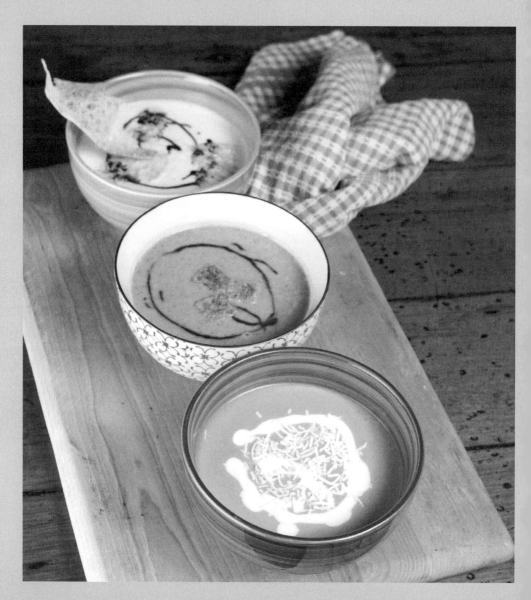

Creamy cauliflower soup with Parmesan croutons

Beautifully smooth and satisfying. If you like cauliflower, you'll love this soup. Ensure that you thoroughly cook the vegetables, and blend for 15 seconds longer than you think for a velvety texture to your puréed soup.

Serves	5-6
Prep time	30 minutes
Cooking time	40 minutes
Carb count	4.8 g per serving

EQUIPMENT

Chopping board, knife, large pot, grater, baking sheet, parchment paper, stand blender or hand blender

INGREDIENTS

Soup

2 onions, sliced

60 g (¼ cup) butter

1 medium head cauliflower, cut into
    smallish pieces

125 ml (½ cup) whole milk

125 ml (½ cup) cream, plus extra as needed

1 liter (1 quart) water, plus extra as needed

salt and pepper to taste

Croutons

50 g (2 oz) Parmesan, Grana Padano, or
    pecorino, grated (6 Tbsp)

METHOD

Preheat the oven to 350°F. Sweat the onions with the butter in the pot over medium heat until they begin to soften. Add the remaining soup ingredients, bring to a boil, and simmer for 25 minutes. Meanwhile, grate the cheese. Line the baking sheet with the parchment paper and scatter the cheese over it in an even layer. Bake for 5-8 minutes, until lightly colored – be careful not to bake for too long, or it will taste a little bitter. Allow to cool and crisp up.

When the soup has had its time, allow it to cool for 10 minutes, then purée it in the blender in batches, or use a hand blender. Adjust the consistency by adding more water and cream, then season to taste. Serve in bowls and crunch over the crispy cheese croutons.

Broccoli & watercress soup with blue-cheese sandwiches

Classic flavors – have you tried them? This soup is also a nice little start to a meal when entertaining. The secret to retaining a vivid green color in the broccoli is to cook it at a continuous boil for 6 minutes before cooling and puréeing.

Serves   about 6
Prep time   25 minutes
Cooking time   20 minutes
Carb count   6.2 g per serving (including
                sandwiches, 0.5 g)

EQUIPMENT

Chopping board, knife, large pot, bowl of cold water, slotted spoon, stand blender or hand blender

INGREDIENTS

2 onions, sliced
100 g (½ cup) butter
1 liter (1 quart) water
2 heads broccoli, cut into florets
100 g (generous 3 cups) watercress (or spinach),
    picked and washed
salt and pepper to taste

Blue-cheese sandwiches

30 g (1 oz) blue cheese, sliced
2 slices Low-Carb Bread (page 156)

METHOD

Sweat the onions in the butter in the pot over medium heat until soft. Add the water and bring to a boil. When the liquid boils, add the broccoli and cook at a rolling (continuous) boil for 6 minutes. Lift the broccoli out of the liquid and cool in the bowl of cold water. Take the liquid off the heat and add the watercress for 30 seconds.

Remove the watercress from the liquid and place in the blender along with the broccoli. Blitz with enough liquid from the pot to enable the soup to blend smoothly. Season with salt and pepper. Serve with blue-cheese sandwiches, cut into neat triangles.

Pumpkin & coconut soup

This soup is light and fragrant. It doesn't have to be a "winter warmer" – it's great any time you have access to pumpkins or hard-shelled squash.

Serves	6–8
Prep time	15 minutes, plus 15 minutes standing time
Cooking time	1 hour
Carb count	12.9 g per serving

EQUIPMENT

Chopping board, knife, large pot, stand blender or hand blender

INGREDIENTS

2 onions, diced

15 g (1 Tbsp) coconut oil (can substitute with olive oil or butter)

1 large cooking pumpkin or winter squash, peeled and diced

2 cloves garlic

1 chili, chopped

375 ml (1½ cups) coconut milk or cream, plus extra to garnish if desired

1 liter (1 quart) water

salt and pepper to taste

1 kaffir lime leaf (optional)

1 stalk lemongrass (optional)

sprinkle of shredded/desiccated coconut to garnish

METHOD

Slowly cook the onion in the oil, and after 5 minutes add in the pumpkin and garlic. Continue to cook for 5 minutes, then add in the remaining ingredients (except the coconut garnish) and allow to simmer for about 45 minutes. Let the soup cool for 15 minutes before puréeing to a smooth consistency. Serve with a sprinkle of shredded coco-nut and a dash of coconut cream.

Create your own salad bar

We cook at home for ourselves and others based on what we would like to eat that night. That's great, but it's time-consuming. In the restaurant, we plan menus that allow for crossover of "prep," to enable efficiencies through bulk-buying discounts and time savings. The following salad recipes are designed to make use of leftovers you might have (or "prepared ahead of time" ingredients), combining them with fresh salad leaves and dressings. By looking ahead and thinking about how we can use leftovers from one meal, we can start to cook with tomorrow's lunch in mind. Allow for extra chicken when making a roast, for example.

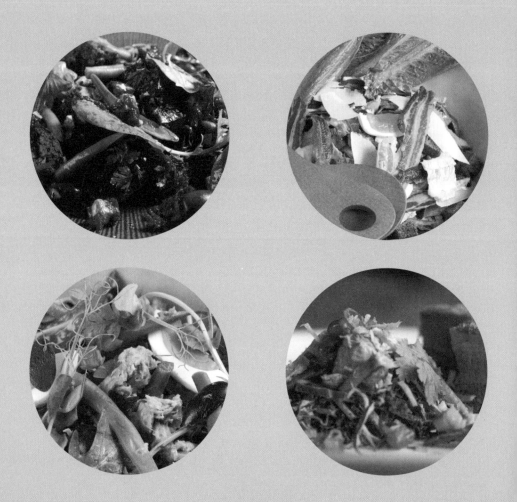

Beets, feta, olives, green beans & arugula

Serves	1–2
Prep time	10 minutes
Carb count	7.1 g per serving

EQUIPMENT

Peeler, chopping board, knife, grater, mixing bowl, pot of boiling water, slotted spoon, bowl of cold water

INGREDIENTS

25 g (¼ small) raw beet
25 g (¼ small) cooked beet (see page 124 for instructions)
15 ml (1 Tbsp) cider vinegar
½ vanilla pod, scraped (optional)
50 g (⅓ cup) green beans, cut into short lengths
25 g (small piece) crumbly feta
10 g (3–4) olives
15 ml (1 Tbsp) French Vinaigrette (page 131)
5 g (4–5) walnuts
5 g (small pinch) diced shallot
salt and pepper to taste
50 g (1½ cups) arugula

METHOD

Peel the raw beet and slice thinly, or grate if preferred. Dice the cooked beet. Mix all of the beet with the cider vinegar and the vanilla (if using) in a bowl large enough to contain the rest of the salad ingredients. Blanch the green beans in the pot of boiling water for 3 minutes, then remove with the slotted spoon and place in the bowl of cold water to cool.

Drain the beans and add to the bowl with the remaining ingredients except the arugula, season well and toss together. Just before serving, stir through half of the arugula. Arrange the salad on a serving plate and top with the remaining arugula.

Roast chicken Caesar salad, soft-boiled eggs & broccoli

Serves	1–2
Prep time	15 minutes
Carb count	4.7 g per serving

EQUIPMENT

Pot of boiling water, chopping board, knives, baking sheet, mixing bowl, scales

INGREDIENTS

1 soft-boiled egg (see page 96 for instructions)
2 slices Low-Carb Bread (page 156), cut into ½-inch cubes
50 g (1 cup) romaine lettuce leaves, washed and drained (iceberg can substitute)
100 g (4 oz) pre-roasted chicken pieces
1 slice pre-cooked bacon
10 g (4 tsp) Parmesan shavings (Grana Padano or pecorino can substitute)
5 g (1 tsp) chopped parsley
50 g (⅓ cup) cooked broccoli
2 anchovies (optional)
30 ml (2 Tbsp) Caesar Dressing (page 130)
salt and pepper to taste

METHOD

Preheat the oven to 350°F. Begin by soft-boiling the eggs (see page 96). Cool the egg by running it under cold water for 5 minutes. Place the bread cubes on the baking sheet and bake in the oven until crunchy, 8–10 minutes.

Chop the lettuce into bite-sized pieces and add to the mixing bowl. Add all the other ingredients except the eggs to the bowl and season. Arrange the salad in a serving bowl, halve or quarter the eggs, and place on top.

Crunchy pulled pork with kaleslaw & tomato salsa

Serves	1–2
Prep time	15 minutes
Carb count	8.6 g per serving

EQUIPMENT

Mixing bowl, chopping board, knife, grater or food processor with grater attachment

INGREDIENTS

100 g (½ cup) Crispy Pork Belly (page 145)
10 ml (2 tsp) Tomato Salsa (page 133)
salt and pepper to taste

Kaleslaw

50 g (¾ cup) picked and washed kale (can substitute with cabbage)
25 g (¼ cup) red cabbage
30 g (½ small) carrot
25 g (¼ small) red onion
30 ml (2 Tbsp) Mayonnaise (page 132)
5 g (1 Tbsp) pumpkin seeds/pepitas
5 g (1½ Tbsp) sunflower seeds
½ chili, sliced (optional)

METHOD

Remove the crispy skin from the pork belly and chop into small pieces. Pull the pork by tearing the meat down the grain (this is much easier when the meat is warm; you can slightly heat the belly if it helps) and combine it with the skin. Add the tomato salsa to the pork and season to taste.

To make the kaleslaw, roughly slice the kale and cabbage and place in the bowl. Grate the carrot into the bowl. Finely slice the red onion and add it to the bowl. Mix in the mayonnaise and seeds and season to finish. Spoon the kaleslaw into a serving bowl and top with the pork. Add fresh chili if desired.

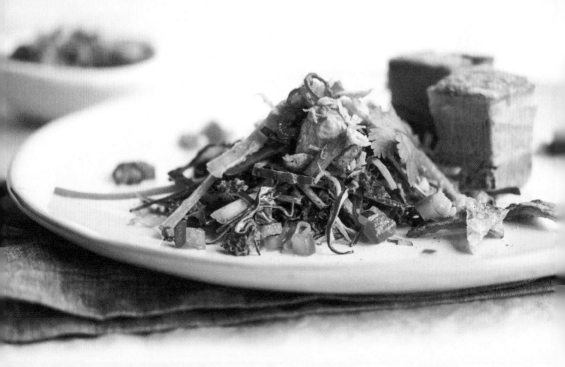

Tuna niçoise

Serves   1-2
Prep time   15 minutes
Cooking time   10 minutes
Carb count   8.9 g per serving

EQUIPMENT

Frying pan, large pot of boiling water, slotted spoon, bowl of cold water, whisk, timer, chopping board, knife

INGREDIENTS

100 g (⅔ cup) fresh tuna (canned works too)
15 ml (1 Tbsp) olive oil if using fresh tuna
15 ml (1 Tbsp) French Vinaigrette (page 131)
salt and pepper to taste
25 g (4-5) green beans, trimmed
50 ml (just under ¼ cup) vinegar
1-2 eggs
100 g (3 cups) mesclun leaves (or other salad greens)
100 g (1 small) tomato, sliced
10 g (3-4) olives, sliced
10 g (2 tsp) chopped parsley

METHOD

If using fresh tuna, sear each side in a hot pan with the olive oil for 20 seconds, leaving the tuna rare in the middle; around 1 minute altogether. Dress the tuna with some of the vinaigrette, season with salt and pepper, and leave to rest.

Blanch the green beans for 3 minutes in the pot of boiling water. Remove the beans using the slotted spoon and place in the bowl of cold water. Add the vinegar to the pot of boiling water and poach the eggs (page 96).

Toss the mesclun leaves with the tomato, drained green beans, olives, parsley, and remaining vinaigrette. Slice the tuna and arrange on top. Serve with the poached eggs. For an alternative, serve with sliced boiled eggs instead.

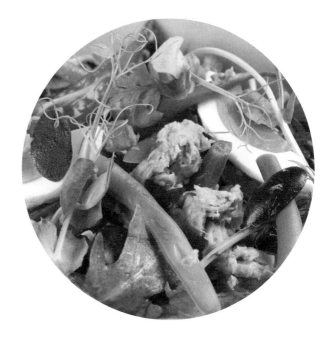

Slow-roasted tomato Caprese salad

Serves   4
Prep time   10 minutes
Cooking time 1 hour
Carb count   9.4 g per serving

EQUIPMENT
Mixing bowls, chopping board, knife,
ovenproof dish

INGREDIENTS
9 tomatoes
45 ml (3 Tbsp) extra-virgin olive oil
sea salt and pepper to taste
50 g (10-12) mushrooms
50 g (2-3 balls) fresh mozzarella
90 g (3 cups) baby spinach, washed and drained
15 g (2 Tbsp) Pesto (page 131)
15 g (2 Tbsp) pine nuts, toasted (see page 100 for
    instructions)
30 g (9-10) olives (optional)
10 g (a few leaves) basil

METHOD
Preheat the oven to 200°F. Halve 8 of the tomatoes.
Place these in a mixing bowl and dress with 1 tablespoon of the olive oil and some salt and pepper. Lay
the tomato halves in the ovenproof dish and slowly
roast in the oven for 1 hour. Meanwhile, panfry
the mushrooms in another tablespoon of olive oil
until tender. After the tomatoes have roasted for
30 minutes, place the mushrooms in the ovenproof
dish alongside the tomatoes and gently re-warm for
30 minutes, until the tomatoes are ready.

Slice the mozzarella and the remaining tomato
and season with sea salt. When the tomatoes and
mushrooms come out of the oven, arrange them on
a plate. Top them with the tomato and mozzarella
slices and sprinkle the baby spinach on top. Dress
the salad by drizzling over the pesto and the other
half of the olive oil, and garnish with the pine nuts,
olives (if using), and basil.

Aromatic beef with Vietslaw

Serves   1-2
Prep time   10 minutes
Carb count   12.3 g per serving

EQUIPMENT
Scales, chopping board, knife, pot of boiling water,
slotted spoon, bowl of cold water, mixing bowl, grater

INGREDIENTS
100 g (4 oz) Panfried Sirloin (page 148) or Slow-
    Cooked Coconut Beef (page 150)

Vietslaw
25 g (4-5) green beans
50 g (½ cup) sliced red cabbage
50 g (½ cup) sliced green cabbage
20 g (¼ small) red or yellow onion, sliced
30 g (½ small) carrot, grated
½ avocado, cut into slices
sliced chili, to taste
5 g (1 tsp) sliced sugar-snap peas
30 ml (2 Tbsp) Lime & Lemongrass Dressing
    (page 130)
5 ml (1 tsp) cider vinegar
salt and pepper to taste

Garnish
15 g (1 Tbsp) toasted cashews (see page 100 for
    instructions)
5 g (1 tsp) chopped cilantro

METHOD
If using the panfried sirloin, slice the sirloin into
¹⁄₁₆-inch slivers. If using the slow-cooked coconut
beef, cut it into bite-sized pieces.

For the Vietslaw, blanch the beans in the pot of
boiling water for 3 minutes, then remove with the
slotted spoon and cool in the bowl of cold water.
Drain. Combine the prepared vegetables in the
mixing bowl with the dressing, the cider vinegar,
and some salt and pepper. Leave to stand for
5 minutes. Arrange the Vietslaw in a serving bowl,
top with the beef, drizzle with some of the juices
from the slaw bowl, and garnish with the cashews
and cilantro.

Grilled chicken skewers, tzatziki & cucumber ribbons

Makes	5 skewers
Prep time	15 minutes
Marinating time	4 hours to overnight (optional)
Cooking time	15 minutes
Carb count	2 g (per skewer and sauce)

EQUIPMENT

Scales, chopping board, knife, bamboo skewers (soak in water for 10 minutes first if using on an outdoor grill), mixing bowl, peeler, melon baller, baking sheet, grater or zester, frying pan or grill pan (or the outdoor grill)

INGREDIENTS

150 g (5 oz) chicken thigh or breast meat

Marinade

20 g (4-5 sprigs) fresh rosemary or thyme
1 clove garlic, crushed
salt and pepper to taste
15 ml (1 Tbsp) olive oil
zest and juice of 1 lemon

Cucumber ribbons and tzatziki

¼ English cucumber (about 75 g/2½ oz)
5 g (2½ tsp) cumin seeds
50 g (¼ cup) unsweetened plain yogurt
    (the thicker the better)
zest and juice of 1 lemon
salt and pepper to taste

METHOD

Cut the chicken into strips and skewer. Make the marinade by combining the ingredients in the mixing bowl. Coat the chicken in the marinade, place the skewers on a plate, and allow the flavors to develop in the fridge for 4 hours, or more if you have time. Grill (or panfry) the chicken skewers over medium heat until they are cooked – they will take a combined time of 5 minutes per side, turning regularly.

Slice the cucumber in half lengthwise and use the melon baller to scoop out the seeds and water, reserving these for adding to the tzatziki. Now cut the cucumber in half crosswise so you have 4 pieces. With a peeler, carefully make thin ribbons of cucumber from 2 of the pieces, reserving the other 2 pieces for later.

Preheat the oven to 350°F. Begin the tzatziki by toasting the cumin seeds on the baking sheet in the oven for 4 minutes. Mix the yogurt with the lemon zest and juice and add in the cumin seeds, salt, and pepper. Stir in a little of the cucumber scrapings you re-served earlier, being careful to stop at the desired consistency (I like a thick, dropping consistency). Mix some tzatziki with the cucumber ribbons and serve alongside the skewers.

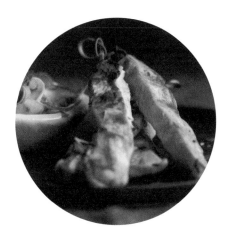

Lamb burger with eggplant bun, feta beet relish & kaleslaw

Replace one cheap, nasty burger bun with some beautiful eggplant and upsize your burger to a happy place. Yes, you may have to forgo the customary eating with your hands here, but at least this way you don't have to contemplate life without burgers!

Serves	3-4
Prep time	15 minutes
Cooking time	15 minutes
Carb count	11.3 g per serving (burger, relish, and kaleslaw)

EQUIPMENT

Scales, grater, bowl, pot with a lid, frying pan, baking sheet

INGREDIENTS

Beet Relish

50 g (½ small) raw beet
15 ml (1 Tbsp) white wine vinegar
15 ml (1 Tbsp) olive oil
15 ml (1 Tbsp) water
50 g (1½ oz) feta, crumbled

500 g (1 lb) ground lamb
1 onion, diced
5 g (1 tsp) ground cumin
1 clove garlic, crushed
salt and pepper to taste
olive oil for cooking
1 eggplant, sliced into ⅜-inch rounds
1 tomato, sliced
20 g (½ oz) cheese per burger (optional)
handful of salad leaves (optional)
100 g (1 cup) Kaleslaw (page 120)

METHOD

Preheat the oven to 350°F. For the relish, peel the beet and grate it into the bowl. Pour the vinegar, olive oil, and water into the pot and bring to a boil. Add the beet to the liquid, cover with a lid, and cook over low heat for 5 minutes. Allow the beet relish to cool completely, then stir through the feta.

Combine the lamb, onion, cumin, garlic, salt, and pepper in a bowl. Form patties the same size as the eggplant slices. Panfry the patties in a little olive oil until lightly colored on both sides and then transfer to the baking sheet. Bake the patties for approximately 6 minutes, depending on size. Meanwhile, clean the frying pan and gently fry the eggplant rounds in some more olive oil for 2 minutes on each side.

When the lamb patties are ready, serve sandwiched between two eggplant slices. Top patties with tomato, cheese, and salad leaves, if desired. Serve burgers with kaleslaw and beet relish on the side. My Oven Fries (page 154) also make a great accompaniment.

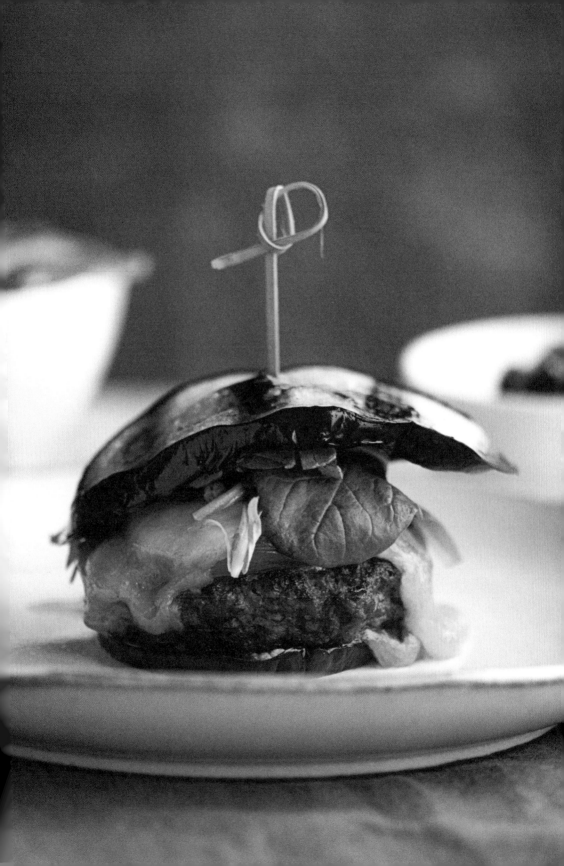

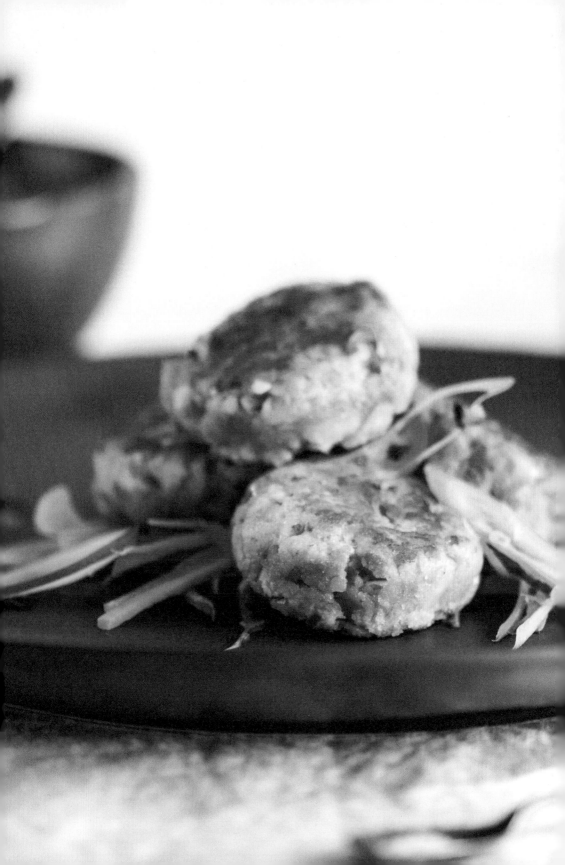

Thai fish cakes

Serve with a light salad for a delicious lunch, or with the dipping sauce as a canapé when entertaining. The cakes can be frozen and pulled out when needed.

Serves	2
Prep time	15 minutes
Cooking time	15 minutes
Carb count	12 g per serving, including dipping sauce

EQUIPMENT

Scales, chopping board, knives, mixing bowl, ovenproof frying pan

EQUIPMENT

Fish cakes

300 g (10 oz) cooked fish (canned salmon or tuna work well, too)

1 onion, diced

1 bell pepper (red or green), diced

5 g (1 tsp) crushed ginger

1 clove garlic, crushed

15 g (1 Tbsp) chopped cilantro

2 eggs, whisked

1 chili, de-seeded and diced (add more or keep the seeds in if you like it spicier)

45 g (⅓ cup) coconut flour

15 ml (1 Tbsp) olive oil

Dipping sauce

30 ml (2 Tbsp) Lime & Lemongrass Dressing (page 130)

5 ml (1 tsp) sweet chili sauce

15 g (1 Tbsp) chopped cilantro

1 green onion, sliced

10 ml (2 tsp) tamari (gluten-free soy sauce)

juice of 1 lime

10 ml (2 tsp) sesame oil

METHOD

Preheat the oven to 350°F. Mix together all the fish cake ingredients except the olive oil, and let the mixture stand for 5 minutes to allow the coconut flour to absorb the moisture. Form patties to your desired size. Fry the patties in the olive oil on both sides and finish in the oven for 3-4 minutes. To make the dipping sauce, simply combine all the ingredients.

Serve the fish cakes with wedges of lime and the dipping sauce on the side. If you want to be as low carb as possible, swap out the dipping sauce for a cilantro and chili mayo (see page 132).

Butter chicken, cauliflower pilau, raita & coconut naan

Impress some friends with this meal for lunch (or dinner). It is best made a day in advance and reheated as you need it. Replacing flour and starchy rice with nutrient-dense ingredients means that this is delicious "health food" – packed with healthy fats and vegetables.

Serves	3-4
Prep time:	30 minutes
Marinating time:	overnight
Cooking time:	45 minutes
Carb count:	18.6 g per serving (including all accompaniments)

EQUIPMENT
Chopping board, knives, food processor, scales, broiler pan, mixing bowl, sieve, frying pan

INGREDIENTS
Marinade
200 g (¾ cup) unsweetened plain yogurt
5 g (2 tsp) cumin seeds
2 cloves garlic
10 g (2-inch piece) fresh ginger, peeled and roughly chopped
10 g (2 Tbsp) tomato paste
10 g (1½ tsp) ground coriander
10 g (1½ tsp) garam masala

500 g (1 lb) chicken thigh or breast, cut into thirds
salt and pepper to taste

Sauce
2 onions, diced
15 g (1 Tbsp) butter
4 whole cloves
1 stick cinnamon (or 5 g/1 tsp ground)
fresh chili or cayenne pepper to taste
30 g (¼ cup) cashew nuts
one 14.5-oz can diced tomatoes
250 ml (1 cup) cream
15 g (1 Tbsp) chopped cilantro

ACCOMPANIMENT 1: COCONUT NAAN
50 g (⅓ cup) coconut flour
pinch of salt
pinch of baking powder
pinch of baking soda
4 eggs, beaten
25 ml (5 tsp) coconut milk
oil for cooking

ACCOMPANIMENT 2: CAULIFLOWER PILAU
200 g (1½ cups) (see variation, page 154)

ACCOMPANIMENT 3: CUCUMBER RAITA
100 g (½ cup) (use tzatziki recipe on page 123, without the cucumber ribbons)

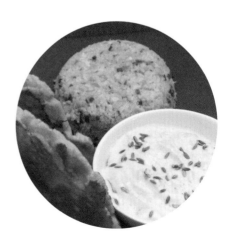

METHOD

Make the marinade by blitzing all the marinade ingredients in the food processor. Marinate the chicken overnight to let the flavors penetrate and the yogurt tenderize the chicken.

The next day, preheat the broiler, then lay the chicken pieces on the broiler pan (reserving the marinade for stirring through the sauce later). Broil until the chicken begins to take on a nice color, about 8 minutes. Season the chicken and transfer to a plate to rest. The chicken will still be undercooked; it will finish cooking in the sauce, ensuring that it is juicy and tender.

Begin the sauce by sweating the onions in the butter in the frying pan over medium heat until lightly browned, then add the spices and cashews and sauté for 2 minutes over medium heat. Add in the tomatoes and allow to reduce for 5 minutes. Remove the cinnamon stick (if used), then transfer the sauce to the food processor and blitz. Push the sauce through the strainer (you may skip this step if you prefer) and add in the chicken, reserved marinade, cream, and cilantro. Bring to a boil and simmer for 4 minutes to finish cooking the chicken and to allow the flavors to combine.

Mix all the ingredients for the coconut naan together and let rest for 5 minutes. Heat a frying pan and add a little oil to the pan. Add the naan mixture, flatten into a large patty, and cook gently for 1-2 minutes on each side, then transfer to a plate. Serve the butter chicken with some or all of the accompaniments for a delicious lunch with friends.

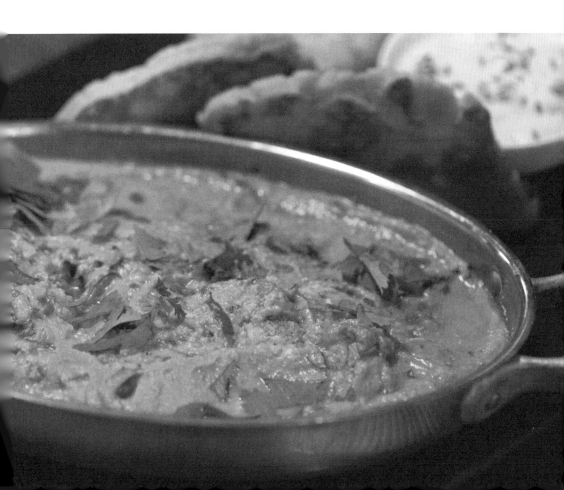

Sauces & dressings

The more sugar, water, and guar gum you can put into a commercially made dressing, the higher your profit margin. For this reason, most store-bought dressings and sauces are not suitable for optimal nutrition, and the LCHF approach avoids them. Most dressings and sauces made traditionally are naturally LCHF and packed with nourishing ingredients. Making a few of the classics ourselves, at home, saves money and adds interest and variety to meals. Our simple recipes show you how easy these kitchen staples are to whip up.

Caesar dressing

The perfect dressing for the Caesar salad on page 119.

Makes	Just over ½ cup
Prep time	15 minutes
Carb count	0.07 g (per Tbsp)

EQUIPMENT

Grater, chopping board, knife, mixing bowl, whisk, storage container

INGREDIENTS

30 ml (2 Tbsp) Mayonnaise (page 132)
10 ml (2 tsp) cider vinegar
50 g (2 oz) hard Italian cheese, grated (6 Tbsp) (Parmesan, Grana Padano, or pecorino, as preferred)
3 anchovies, chopped
2 cloves garlic, crushed
60 ml (¼ cup) water
15 g (1 Tbsp) chopped soft herbs (parsley or chives work well)
salt and pepper to taste

METHOD

In the bowl, whisk together all the ingredients and season to taste. Transfer to a jar or container with a lid and keep refrigerated for up to 1 week.

Lime & lemongrass dressing

Kept in the fridge, this amazing dressing will last for a month. It is easily halved if you don't have a large family.

Makes	1 quart
Prep time	15 minutes
Carb count	0.4 g (per Tbsp)

EQUIPMENT

Chopping board, knife, blender or food processor, fine-mesh sieve, clean storage container

INGREDIENTS

300 g (10 oz) fresh ginger, peeled and roughly chopped (2 cups)
200 g (7 oz) lemongrass, roughly chopped (1½ cups)
100 g (about 3) chilies, de-seeded and roughly chopped
zest and juice of 6 limes
30 g (1 oz/1 cup) kaffir lime leaves (optional)
8 cloves garlic
60 ml (¼ cup) sesame oil
90 ml (6 Tbsp) fish sauce
100 g (4 cups) picked mint leaves
100 g (4 cups) picked cilantro leaves
375 ml (1½ cups) water

METHOD

Place all the ingredients in the blender or food processor and blitz for 20-30 seconds. Strain through the sieve, and then bottle the dressing in a suitable container. Keep in the fridge and shake before use, as the layers will separate naturally.

French vinaigrette

The secret to this vinaigrette is to allow some time for the flavors to develop. We give it three weeks to mature.

Makes	2 cups
Prep time	8 minutes
Carb count	0.1 g (per Tbsp)

EQUIPMENT
Mixing bowl, whisk or food processor, measuring cup, scales, clean jar or bottle

INGREDIENTS
85 ml (⅓ cup) cider vinegar or white wine vinegar
15 ml (1 Tbsp) Dijon mustard
300 ml (1¼ cups) olive oil
2 cloves garlic
15 g (3 sprigs) fresh thyme
15 g (3 sprigs) fresh rosemary
5 g (1 tsp) peppercorns
2 bay leaves
10 g (2 tsp) salt

METHOD
Mix the vinegar with the mustard. Slowly whisk the oil into the vinegar-and-mustard mix until fully incorporated. Add the rest of the ingredients and bottle. You can skip the slow-whisking part and simply mix all the ingredients together, but the vinaigrette will be split; just remember to shake the vinaigrette thoroughly before use. Alternatively, use a food processor to combine the vinegar, mustard, and oil and then add the rest of the ingredients.

Pesto

Makes enough for a small jar that will keep you going for a week plus.

Makes	one ¾-cup jar
Prep time	15 minutes
Carb count	0.3 g (per Tbsp)

EQUIPMENT
Grater, food processor or hand blender or jug blender, clean jar

INGREDIENTS
50 g (2 oz) hard Italian cheese
    (Parmesan, Grana Padano, or pecorino, as
    preferred)
100 g (4 cups) picked basil leaves
30 g (¼ cup) toasted pine nuts (see page 100
    for instructions)
15 g (2 Tbsp) cashew nuts
1 clove garlic
50 g (1½ cups) arugula
125 ml (½ cup) olive oil or extra-virgin olive oil
15 ml (1 Tbsp) water
salt and pepper to taste

METHOD
Grate the cheese into the appropriate bowl or container for the blending machine you are using. Add the remaining ingredients except the oil and water. Begin to blitz the ingredients and steadily pour in the oil until the pesto begins to look creamy. Add a splash of water to help the pesto stay creamy, and give a last blend as you season to taste. Transfer to a suitable jar or container. Best used within 2 weeks.

Mayonnaise

Easy to make, lasts a week and a half in the fridge, and forms the base of a range of dressings and flavored mayos. This is a great recipe to introduce to your kitchen. It will make a large jar, so you may want to sterilize a jar for this by washing it in a dishwasher.

Makes	one 20-oz jar
Prep time	15 minutes
Carb count	0.03 g (per Tbsp)

EQUIPMENT

Mixing bowl and whisk, or food processor, measuring cup, airtight container or jar

INGREDIENTS

3 eggs

15 ml (1 Tbsp) mustard (Dijon, whole-grain, or English as preferred)

15 ml (1 Tbsp) cider vinegar

salt and pepper to taste

500 ml (2 cups) olive oil

15 ml (1 Tbsp) water (only if necessary)

METHOD

In a restaurant kitchen, we have the luxury of using a food processor to make our mayo. If you have one, I strongly recommend using it. Secondly, I like to use regular olive oil for making mayonnaise, as it is a bit less intrusive than extra-virgin olive oil - but you're the boss, so experiment and see what you prefer. I also recommend using vinegar (acetic acid) instead of lemon (citric acid) to sharpen the mayo, as I find the lemon reacts with the olive oil to produce a bitter flavor. Lastly, I was taught to use whole eggs and I have never found any problems with this. It increases yield and reduces wasted egg whites.

Crack the eggs into the mixing bowl or the bowl of your food processor. Add in the mustard, vinegar, and seasoning. Begin to whisk (or start the blades running) and slowly trickle in the olive oil. As the mixture begins to thicken (when approximately half of the oil has been mixed in), you can increase the speed at which you add the oil. Once the oil is incorporated, adjust the thickness with some water if necessary and season to taste. Transfer the mayonnaise to a suitably sized airtight container and keep in the fridge for up to 3 days.

This mayo forms the base of many other dressings and sauces: add chopped capers, gherkins, shallots, and herbs for a tartar sauce. Or try adding some finely chopped chili and cilantro - goes beautifully with our Thai Fish Cakes (page 127).

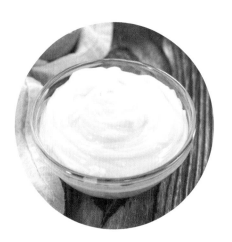

Guacamole

Where LCHF cooking is concerned, avocados are an essential staple ingredient, full of fat and flavor and adding a wonderful richness to dishes.

Serves	6–8
Prep time	15 minutes
Carb count	0.1 g (per Tbsp)

EQUIPMENT

Chopping board, knife, mixing bowl, or a hand or stand blender (if doing the purée method)

INGREDIENTS

3 ripe avocados
1 red chili, finely chopped (de-seed it for less heat)
juice of 2 limes
25 g (2 Tbsp) chopped cilantro
½ clove garlic, grated
salt and pepper to taste
30 ml (2 Tbsp) extra-virgin olive oil (or 60 ml/
    ¼ cup for a smoother, purée-style guacamole)
30 ml (2 Tbsp) water (for a smoother, purée-style
    guacamole)

METHOD

If making the guacamole by hand, start by chopping the avocados as small or as large as you like. Add the remaining ingredients and season to taste. It will keep for 1–2 days only.

I like a refined, purée consistency to my guacamole, almost like an avocado aïoli. To do this, begin by blitzing the avocado in the food processor with all the ingredients except the oil. When the mixture is smooth and mixing nicely, start pouring the oil into the moving mixture in the style of making a mayonnaise; the resultant purée will be smooth, thick, and incredible. Give it a go, we love it!

Tomato salsa

In summer, instead of cooking the salsa I leave the combined ingredients, covered, outside in direct sunlight for an hour before I need them; the sun's heat takes the rawness out of the veggies without destroying their vibrant flavor or texture.

Serves	3–4
Prep time	15 minutes
Cooking time	20 minutes, plus 15 minutes standing time
Carb count	0.4 g (per Tbsp)

EQUIPMENT

Chopping board, knife, mixing bowl (not aluminium), pot

INGREDIENTS

2 ripe tomatoes, diced
1 red onion, diced
¼ clove garlic
15 g (1 Tbsp) chopped cilantro
juice of 2 limes
1 bell pepper (color of your preference), diced
1 green onion, finely sliced
1–2 (depending on preference) chilies, de-seeded
    and finely chopped
15 ml (1 Tbsp) vinegar
20 ml (4 tsp) extra-virgin olive oil
celery salt (optional), to taste
salt and pepper to taste

METHOD

Mix all the ingredients together in the bowl to allow the salt and vinegar to draw liquid from the salsa. After 15 minutes, strain the liquid into the pot with about one-quarter of the mixture. Bring to a boil and simmer for 10 minutes, until it has reduced considerably. This step activates the natural pectin in the tomato. Once the cooked mixture has cooled, stir it through the remaining salsa and refrigerate. The pectin will help to thicken the salsa. Keep refrigerated for up to 1 week.

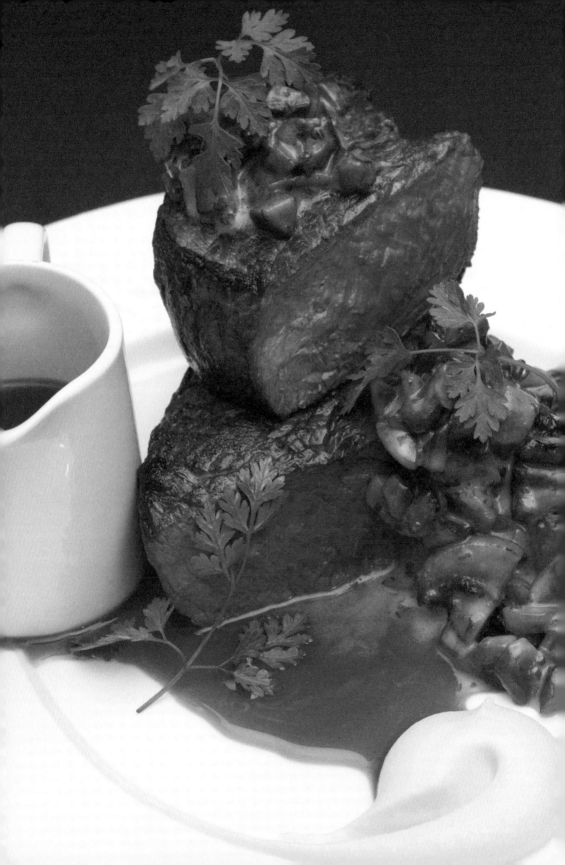

Dinner

These recipes will hopefully help to show you how to cook dinner for yourself and others. Some of the recipes I've practically lifted from the restaurant's kitchen, so I hope you have a go at them and share them with your friends and family. Remember to make use of your butcher for portioning your meat. You will likely want to use between four and five ounces raw weight of meat per person, but this varies based on your personal requirements. Use your discretion and let the butcher help, or use food labels on supermarket meat packs as a guide.

It's a good idea to buy larger quantities of meat and salmon when they're on special, then divide them up into portions and freeze what you don't need right away (pin-bone the salmon and wrap everything tightly in plastic wrap before freezing). Defrost portions as you need them over the next few weeks.

Winner, winner, chicken dinner!
(Roast chicken) with green vegetables & rich roast gravy

Who doesn't love roast chicken on a Sunday? The leftover meat and vegetables (if any) are perfect to start off the next week's lunches.

Serves	4
Prep time	20 minutes
Cooking time	1 hour 40 minutes
Carb count	9.2 g per serving, including sides

EQUIPMENT

Knives, large roasting dish, large pot of boiling salted water, medium pot, colander

INGREDIENTS

3 onions, peeled and halved
3 carrots, roughly chopped
2 parsnips, roughly chopped
one 3½- to 4-lb free-range chicken
50 g (¼ cup) butter
salt and pepper to taste
10 g (2 tsp) chopped fresh rosemary
10 g (2 tsp) chopped fresh thyme
10 g (2 tsp) chopped fresh oregano
2 whole bulbs garlic, cut in half
2 lemons, halved
100 g (5 slices) bacon
60 ml (¼ cup) cream

Sides

300 g (3 cups) Brussels sprouts (or green beans or
    asparagus, depending on season), trimmed
1 head broccoli, cut into florets
15 g (1 Tbsp) butter

METHOD

Preheat the oven to 350°F. Lay the prepared vegetables (onions, carrots, parsnips) in the roasting dish and place the chicken on top. Smear the chicken with the butter and season well. Place the herbs, garlic, and halved lemons inside the chicken cavity. Take the bacon and fold it in half lengthwise. Tuck the bacon in between the chicken and the vegetables to protect the bacon from excessive cooking. Put the dish in the preheated oven for approximately 80 minutes.

After 30 minutes, stir the vegetables roasting with the chicken. Spoon over some of the cooking juices to baste the chicken. When the 80 minutes is up, remove the chicken and the bacon from the dish and sit them on a large plate. Carefully remove the herbs, lemon, and garlic from the cavity and return them to the vegetables in the dish to go back in the oven for another 20 minutes. Cover the chicken and bacon with tin foil and a kitchen towel and let the chicken rest for at least 20 minutes.

Cook the Brussels sprouts in the large pot of water for 3 minutes, then add in the broccoli and cook for a further 3 minutes – if using green beans or asparagus, cook at the same time as the broccoli, for 3 minutes only. Drain the vegetables in the colander and return them to the now-empty pot. Add in the butter and some salt and cracked pepper, stir together, and then leave in the pot to stay warm.

Take the roasted vegetables out of the oven. Arrange the vegetables on a large serving dish and pour the roasting juices into the medium pot. Add a little water to the roasting dish and gently scrape off the sediment on the bottom - pour this into the pot with the roasting juices. Begin to heat the juices over high heat to reduce. Transfer the chicken to a chopping board and pour any juices into the gravy pot. Carve the chicken as you like, and arrange on the serving dish beside the vegetables and bacon. Add the cream to the roasting juices and continue to boil for 2 minutes. The result is a deliciously rich sauce/gravy with all the goodness of the roasted chicken and vegetables.

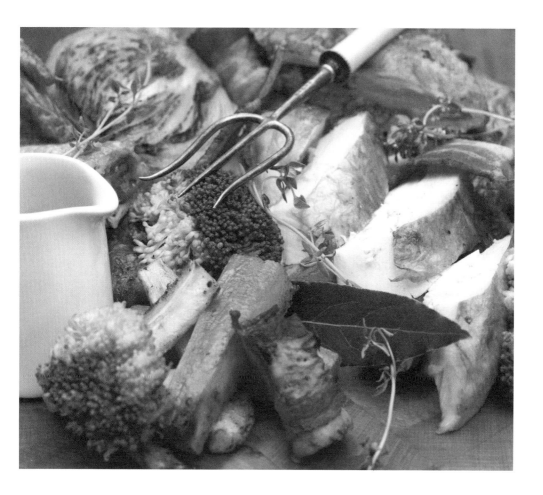

Smoked fish pie with peas & prawns

A guaranteed winner and always great for leftovers. It freezes really well, too. You can easily substitute the fish for others you may have or really like – salmon is another excellent option.

Serves	3-4
Prep time	15 minutes
Cooking time	45 minutes
Carb count	9.6 g per serving

EQUIPMENT

Chopping board, knives, medium pot, scales, baking dish, large pot of boiling salted water, colander

INGREDIENTS

1-2 onions, diced
1-2 carrots, diced
1 rib celery, diced
100 g (4 oz; 15-20) mushrooms, diced
30 g (2 Tbsp) butter
250 ml (1 cup) cream
1 bay leaf (optional)
zest of ½ lemon (optional)
150 g (5 oz) smoked fish, cut into bite-sized pieces
250 g (8 oz) white fish (sole, cod, or similar),
      cut into bite-sized pieces
30 g (2 Tbsp) frozen peas
100 g (4 oz) frozen prawns
1 recipe Creamy Mash (page 153)
50 g (1½ oz) cheddar, grated (6 Tbsp)
3-4 soft-boiled eggs (see page 96 for instructions);
      1 per person
100 g (1 cup) asparagus or broccoli or
      green beans
15 g (1 Tbsp) butter
salt and pepper to taste

METHOD

Preheat the oven to 350°F. Sauté the onions, carrots, celery, and mushrooms (if using) in the pot with the butter. Add in the cream, bay leaf, and lemon zest (if using). Bring to a boil and simmer to reduce for 5 minutes. Add in the fish and continue to simmer for 3 minutes. Add in the peas and prawns and transfer to the baking dish. Allow the mix to cool in the dish for 20 minutes, as this will make putting the mash top on easier.

Starting from the edges (like a jigsaw), spoon the mash into the dish, working your way around the dish until you have a border of mash. Fill in the rest of the dish with the mash spoonful by spoonful until the dish is covered over, and then spread to cover the entire filling. Sprinkle on the grated cheese and bake for 30 minutes.

Shortly before the pie is ready, prepare the eggs and cook the green vegetables in the large pot of water for 3 minutes. Drain the vegetables in the colander and return them to the now-empty pot. Add in the butter and some salt and cracked pepper. Serve the pie piping hot along with the buttered green vegetables and soft-boiled eggs.

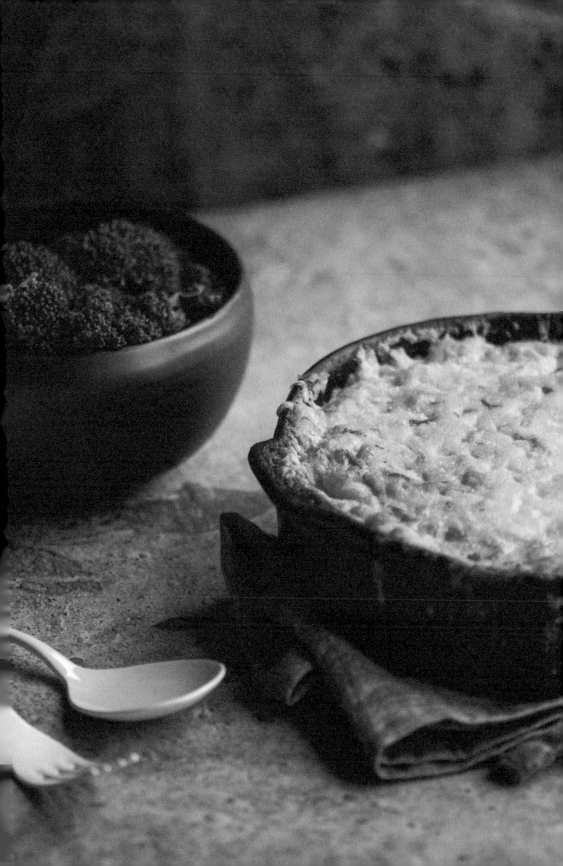

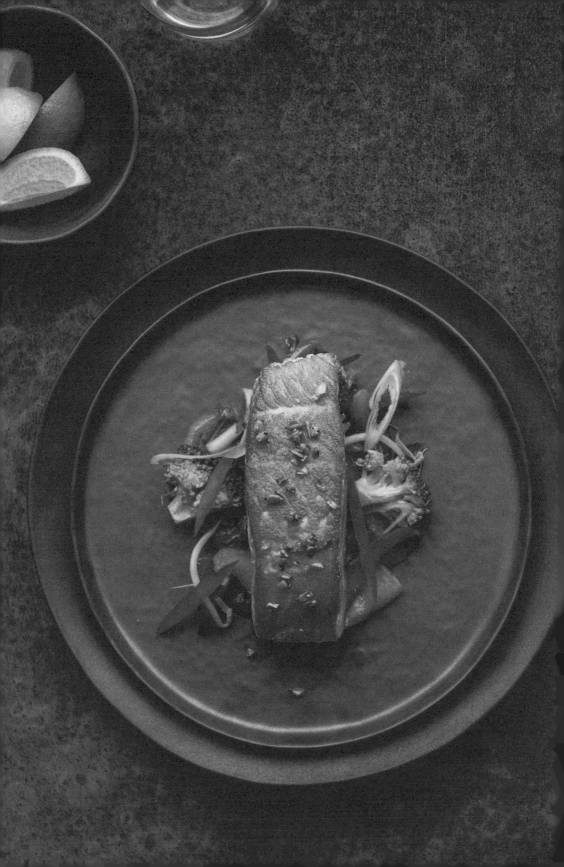

Sesame-roasted salmon with stir-fried vegetables

Oily, soft salmon with a crispy skin is such a treat. Serve with a simple stir-fry for a fantastic meal in under fifteen minutes.

Serves 4
Prep time 30 minutes
Cooking time 12 minutes
Carb count 6.1 g per serving

EQUIPMENT

Chopping board, knives, fish slice or spatula, ovenproof frying pan or ordinary frying pan plus baking sheet (preheated in the oven), large wok or frying pan

INGREDIENTS

Four 120–150 g (4- to 5-oz) fillets salmon, skin on
15 ml (1 Tbsp) tamari (gluten-free soy sauce)
5 ml (1 tsp) sesame oil
5 g (1½ tsp) sesame seeds

Stir-fried vegetables

20 ml (4 tsp) olive oil
1-2 onions, sliced
1-2 bell peppers (any color), sliced
1-2 bok choy, sliced
100 g (4 oz) broccoli, florets separated
  and cut in half
100 g (1 cup) bean sprouts
100 g (1 cup) sugar-snap peas, sliced
50 g (10-12) mushrooms, sliced
10 g (2-inch piece) fresh ginger, peeled and chopped
1 clove garlic, chopped
15 ml (1 Tbsp) tamari (gluten-free soy sauce)
5 ml (1 tsp) sesame oil
pinch of Chinese five spice (optional)

To serve

15 g (2 Tbsp) toasted nuts (optional;
  see page 100 for instructions)
½ green onion, sliced (optional)

METHOD

Preheat the oven to 400°F. Slice the vegetables for the stir-fry. Make a marinade for the salmon by combining the tamari and sesame oil, and gently turn the fish in it; leave to stand for 1 minute. With a paper towel, wipe the moisture from the skin of the salmon and coat the flesh side with the sesame seeds. Heat the ovenproof pan on medium-high heat and put the salmon in skin side down. Put a bit of pressure on the salmon to ensure that the skin makes good contact with the pan. After 3-4 minutes, the skin should start to get crispy. Transfer the ovenproof pan to the oven (or transfer the fish to the preheated baking sheet) and cook for 4 minutes.

While the fish is in the oven, heat the wok or large frying pan and add the olive oil. Add all the vegetables, including the ginger and garlic, and stir-fry for 2 minutes. Add in the tamari, sesame oil, and five spice – as the liquid boils away, the vegetables should cook to a soft, but crunchy, finish. Remove the fish from the oven, allow it to rest for 2 minutes and then pour any juices into the stir-fried vegetables. Serve the salmon on top of the vegetables, or with Zucchini Noodles (page 153) as an alternative. Sprinkle with nuts and some sliced green onion, if desired.

Beef & chicken-liver meatballs with caponata & pine nuts

Italian and French kids grow up eating offal prepared in the most delicious ways; I grew up wondering what the odd, unappetizing smell coming from the kitchen was (sorry, Mum). If you are a bit unsure about offal, this recipe is a great entry point to overcoming that fear! Ask your butcher to grind some chicken liver through the ground beef in a ratio of three parts beef to one part chicken liver. Liver adds a lovely dimension of flavor and is regarded as a culinary multivitamin.

Serves	3-4
Prep time	30 minutes, plus 15 minutes cooling time
Cooking time	1 hour
Carb count	11 g per serving

EQUIPMENT
Chopping boards, knives, food processor, 2 frying pans, mixing bowls

INGREDIENTS
Meatballs
300 g (10 oz) ground beef
100 g (4 oz) chicken livers
1 onion, diced
1 clove garlic, crushed
15 ml (1 Tbsp) olive oil
5 g (1 tsp) chopped fresh thyme
5 g (1 tsp) chopped fresh rosemary
5 g (1 tsp) dried oregano
15 ml (1 Tbsp) tomato paste
15 g (1 Tbsp) chopped fresh parsley
salt and pepper to taste
1 egg, beaten

Tomato sauce
1 onion, diced
1 clove garlic, chopped
15 ml (1 Tbsp) olive oil
100 ml (one-fourth of a 14.5-oz can) canned diced tomatoes
15 g (1 Tbsp) roughly chopped fresh basil

Caponata
1 eggplant, roughly diced
30 ml (2 Tbsp) olive oil
1 red onion, diced
1 bell pepper (any color), diced
10 g (2 tsp) capers, chopped
20 g (7-8) olives, roughly chopped
salt and pepper to taste
15 ml (1 Tbsp) white wine
125 ml (½ cup) water
15 g (1 Tbsp) tomato paste

To serve
15 g (2 Tbsp) toasted pine nuts (see page 100 for instructions)

METHOD

To make the meatballs, take half the ground meat and all the liver and pulse together in a food processor until the meat has an even texture. Sauté the onion and garlic in the olive oil and add in the thyme, rosemary, and oregano. Cook for 2 minutes over medium heat, then add in the tomato paste and cook for 1 minute. Take off the heat, stir through the parsley, and season. Transfer the mix to a bowl and cool for 15 minutes before adding in the ground meats and beaten egg. Mix everything well, then take a small amount and cook it in a frying pan to check the seasoning. You shouldn't need any oil, but add a little if the mixture starts to stick. Adjust the seasoning and herbs, and repeat until you are happy with the mix. Cover and rest the meatball mix in the fridge for 30 minutes.

Wipe out the frying pan and make the simple tomato sauce by frying the onion and garlic in the oil for 1 minute over medium heat. Add in the tomatoes and cook over low heat for 10 minutes.

Start the caponata in the other frying pan. Fry the eggplant in the olive oil until it begins to color. Add the onion, bell pepper, capers, and olives and continue to fry for 1-2 minutes. Season with salt and pepper. Add the white wine, water, and tomato paste and cook over medium heat for 5 minutes. Take the caponata off the heat and cover.

Take the meatball mix from the fridge and form it into balls about the size of golf balls. Fry the meatballs for 3-4 minutes, until they take on a bit of color, then pour over the tomato sauce and simmer for 10 minutes. Once the meatballs are cooked through, stir through the basil and pour over the caponata sauce. Garnish with the pine nuts and some chopped fresh herbs, if desired.

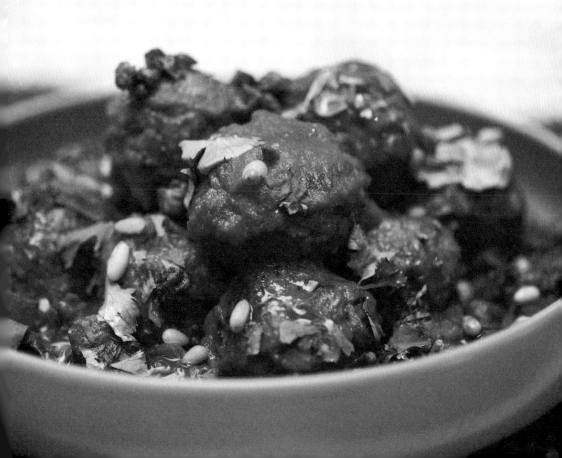

Wine-braised beef stew with mushrooms & onions

Stews develop and improve in flavor over many hours, so they are ideal to prepare on a not-so-lazy Sunday. They freeze perfectly and are always a family favorite.

Serves 4
Prep time 15 minutes
Cooking time 1½ hours minimum
Carb count 5.5 g per serving

EQUIPMENT

Chopping boards, knives, large casserole dish with lid, frying pan

INGREDIENTS

100 g (12) pearl onions, peeled
50 g (10-12) mushrooms, halved
1-2 onions, diced
100 g (1 medium) carrot, roughly diced
50 g (½ small) parsnip, roughly diced
500 g (1 lb) flat iron steak, diced (shoulder or chuck steak work well, too)
1-2 sprigs thyme
4 cloves garlic, chopped
165 ml (⅔ cup) red wine
250 ml (1 cup) chicken stock or water
5 g (1 tsp) tomato paste
10 ml (2 tsp) Dijon mustard (English or whole-grain is fine, too)
salt and pepper to taste

METHOD

Preheat the oven to 325°F. Prepare the vegetables and place in the casserole dish. Heat the frying pan and brown the meat in batches without crowding (you shouldn't need any oil), then add it to the casserole dish with all the other ingredients. Put the lid on the dish and cook in the oven for at least 1½ hours, up to 3 hours at the most (any longer and the meat will break up). If you have a fancy oven or a slow cooker, you can set it to turn off after 3 hours and put the stew in before leaving for work.

Serve the stew with some Creamy Mash (page 153) and green vegetables.

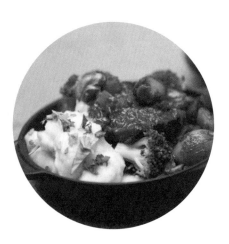

Crispy pork belly with stir-fried vegetables

*Once you get the pork belly crunchy, it stays crunchy. So, if you like to throw some crunchy diced pork into
a salad, cooking enough of this so you have leftovers means that tomorrow's lunch is waiting for you in the fridge.*

Serves	4
Prep time	20 minutes
Cooking time	1½ hours
Carb count	7.1 g per serving, including vegetables

EQUIPMENT

Chopping boards, knives, broiler pan or wire rack set in a baking pan, pot, hand blender

INGREDIENTS

1 kg (2¼ lb) free-range pork belly
15 ml (1 Tbsp) tamari (gluten-free soy sauce)
5 ml (1 tsp) sesame oil
5 g (1 tsp) Chinese five spice
2 whole bulbs garlic, halved
500 ml (2 cups) water
125 ml (½ cup) white wine

Sauce

250 ml (1 cup) cooking liquid from the pork
45 ml (3 Tbsp) tamari (gluten-free soy sauce)
15 ml (1 Tbsp) fish sauce
10 g (2-inch piece) fresh ginger, peeled and crushed
50 g (⅓ cup) black sesame seeds

1 recipe Stir-Fried Vegetables (page 141)

METHOD

Preheat the oven to 425°F. Rub the pork belly flesh with the tamari, sesame oil, and five spice – being careful not to get it on the skin, as it might burn. Place the garlic on the broiler pan or wire rack, place the pork on top of the garlic, skin side up, and roast them in the hot oven for 12-15 minutes. Then reduce the temperature to 350°F, and add the water and wine to the tray beneath the pork. Continue cooking for 1-1½ hours, until the pork meat can be pulled apart easily. Transfer the pork to a chopping board to rest.

To make the sauce, measure the pork cooking liquid into the pot, bring to a boil, and reduce by two-thirds. Push the now-soft garlic cloves out of their skins and into the liquid, and add the tamari, fish sauce, and ginger. Quickly blitz the sauce with a hand blender to purée the garlic and help emulsify the fats with the liquids, which will thicken the sauce slightly. Stir in the sesame seeds and transfer to a pouring jug. Prepare the stir-fried vegetables as on page 141.

Lift the crispy skin off the pork and cut pieces of the meat to serve. Crunch the skin over the meat and serve with the vegetables and sesame-seed sauce.

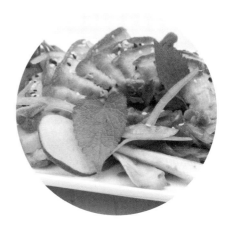

Olive-oil-poached lamb sirloin with beet, roast pumpkin & cumin labneh

This recipe is a bit more complicated, but the results are stunning, especially the pairing of the lamb with the labneh (spiced yogurt that's been hung to let the whey drain off). Give it a go and impress your friends – and yourself. It's really handy to have a probe thermometer when cooking this dish.

Serves	4
Prep time	35 minutes plus hanging the labneh
Cooking time	1½ hours
Carb count	11.8 g per serving

EQUIPMENT

2 bowls, cheesecloth or thin kitchen towel, large sieve, pot of boiling salted water, scales, chopping board, knives, roasting dish, large empty pot, temperature probe, frying pan

INGREDIENTS

Labneh

250 ml (1 cup) unsweetened plain yogurt
10 ml (2 tsp) lemon juice
3 g (½ tsp) ground cumin
salt and pepper to taste

Accompaniments

150 g (5 oz; 1 medium) beet
200 g (7 oz) pumpkin or winter squash, sliced into
        8 wedges
15 ml (1 Tbsp) olive oil
salt and pepper to taste

Lamb

600 g (1⅓ lb) lamb sirloin
250 ml (1 cup) olive oil
1–2 sprigs rosemary
10 peppercorns
1 bay leaf
10 g (2 tsp) salt
1 whole bulb garlic, halved

METHOD

Mix the ingredients for the labneh together in one of the bowls. Line the sieve with the cheesecloth or kitchen towel and scrape the contents of the bowl out into the lined sieve. Tie the edges of the cloth together and leave inside the sieve with the other bowl underneath to collect the liquid, placing it all in the fridge. The longer it hangs, the thicker the labneh – up to a whole day for a soft-cheese consistency.

Preheat the oven to 350°F. Boil the whole beet in the pot of seasoned water until tender (a medium beet will take up to 45 minutes). Toss the wedges of pumpkin in the oil and seasoning and roast in the oven for 30 minutes.

While the vegetables are cooking, place the lamb in the large pot and submerge it in the oil. Add the rosemary, peppercorns, bay leaf, salt, and garlic and heat until the oil is hot to the touch but not bubbling at all. Put the temperature probe into the meat and cook to the degree you like – I find 136°F to be ideal for the lamb; this will take almost 1½ hours.

Once the beet is cooked, remove it from the water and cool in some cold water for 2 minutes to make it easier to handle when peeling. Peel the beet by pushing its skin off (you might want to wear gloves) and dice as small or as chunky as you like. Transfer the beet to the oven alongside the pumpkin to stay warm. Once the pumpkin is soft, turn off the oven and leave the door ajar.

Heat the frying pan and color the cooked lamb on all sides, giving the skin side about 4 minutes to render and crisp up. Transfer the lamb to a cutting board and let it rest for 2–3 minutes (the slow poaching means that the lamb needs very little resting time).

Serve the beet and pumpkin onto plates, carve the lamb, and arrange the meat next to the vegetables along with some of the labneh.

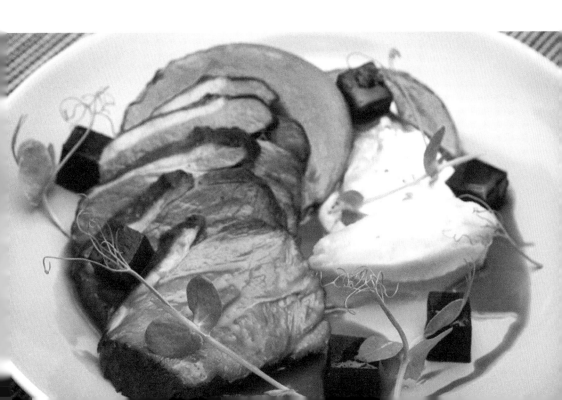

Panfried sirloin with celery root purée, truffled spinach, kale & roast mushroom fondue

In French cuisine, lean cuts of meat were traditionally paired with rich sauces and garnishes. This is how cooks intuitively found the best way to amplify the lovely soft texture of steak or fish and give it a higher fat content to satisfy the diner. This little dish will definitely impress your dinner date, and it's actually pretty simple.

Serves	4
Prep time	40 minutes
Cooking time	40 minutes
Carb count	5.2 g per serving

EQUIPMENT

Chopping boards, knives, small pot, large pot of boiling salted water, colander, 2 frying pans, mixing bowl

INGREDIENTS

Celery root purée
1 onion, chopped
15 g (1 Tbsp) butter
200 g (7 oz) celery root, peeled and chopped
60 ml (¼ cup) cream
5 g (1 tsp) chopped fresh thyme
170 ml (⅔ cup) chicken stock or water

Mushroom fondue
125 ml (½ cup) Hollandaise Sauce (page 109)
100 g (4 oz; 15-20) mushrooms, diced
15 g (1 Tbsp) butter
10 g (2 tsp) sliced fresh chives
5 g (1 tsp) chopped fresh tarragon

Accompaniments
150 g (5 oz) kale leaves
150 g (5 oz) spinach leaves
30 g (2 Tbsp) butter
10 ml (2 tsp) truffle oil (optional)

Sirloin
5 ml (1 tsp) coconut oil, olive oil, or
    clarified butter for cooking
four 150-g (5-oz) beef sirloin steaks (ask your
    butcher or check the weight on
    the label)
10 g (2 tsp) butter
1 sprig thyme
1 clove garlic, crushed
salt and pepper to taste

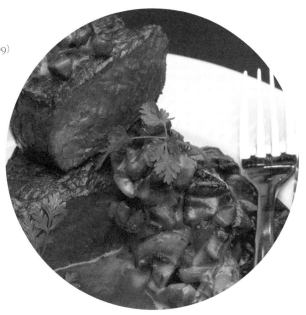

METHOD

To make the celery root purée, sweat the chopped onion with the butter in the small pot over medium heat. Add in the celery root, cream, thyme, and chicken stock or water. Bring to a boil and simmer for 20–25 minutes, until the celery root is soft. Allow to cool slightly, and then blend until smooth.

Make the hollandaise sauce and keep covered. Blanch the kale in the pot of boiling water for 2 minutes, drain, and leave to cool in a colander.

To prepare the sirloin, heat the oil or clarified butter over medium heat and panfry the sirloin, turning every 30 seconds for even cooking. Once the steak is colored and has had about 2 minutes in the pan, add in the butter, thyme, garlic, and seasoning. Continue to cook for 2 minutes – turning every 30 seconds – then remove from the pan and allow to rest for 5 minutes. This method will result in a rare to medium-rare steak that is on the point of releasing its juices. If you prefer your steak more well done, increase the cooking time in 1-minute increments until you find your perfect point.

To make the mushroom fondue, sauté the mushrooms in the butter in the second frying pan until golden. Transfer to a mixing bowl, season, and add the chives and tarragon. Spoon in some of the hollandaise to bind the mushrooms together.

Sauté the spinach in the butter and then stir through the blanched kale and the truffle oil (if using).

Arrange the vegetables on a serving plate. Slice the meat on a shallow angle and season the inside before transferring to the plate. Spoon some celery root purée next to the beef and finish by pouring some mushroom fondue over the meat.

Slow-cooked coconut beef with squash purée, cucumber & cilantro salad

Rich and satisfying, but somehow also light and interesting, beef cheek cooks down to a sticky, gelatinous hunk of meat. If it's unavailable, I recommend flat iron steak.

Serves	4
Prep time	15 minutes
Cooking time	2 hours
Carb count	8.7 g per serving

EQUIPMENT
Frying pan, casserole dish, chopping board, knives, small pot, blender, larger pot, mixing bowl

INGREDIENTS

Beef

500 g (1 lb) beef cheek or flat iron steak
300 ml (1¼ cups) coconut milk
500 ml (2 cups) water
2 kaffir lime leaves (optional)
2 fresh chilies, halved
2 sticks lemongrass, bashed
50 g (5-inch piece) fresh ginger, peeled and
   chopped
salt and pepper to taste

Pumpkin purée

15 ml (1 Tbsp) olive oil
1 onion, sliced
200 g (⅓ small) winter squash or baking pumpkin,
   peeled, de-seeded, and roughly chopped
5 g (1-inch piece) fresh ginger, peeled and chopped
250 ml (1 cup) water

Cucumber & cilantro salad

100 g (½ small) cucumber, cut into ribbons as on
   page 123)
15 g (2 Tbsp) toasted cashew nuts (see page 100
   for instructions)
15 g (2 Tbsp) sesame seeds
30 ml (2 Tbsp) Lime & Lemongrass Dressing
   (page 130)
30 g (⅓ cup) bean sprouts
15 g (1 Tbsp) chopped cilantro

METHOD

Preheat the oven to 325°F. Sear the beef in a hot frying pan (you shouldn't need any oil) and transfer it to the casserole dish. Add the rest of the ingredients for the beef to the dish, reserving a quarter of the aromatics (lime leaves, lemongrass, ginger) for later to add freshness back into the sauce after the long cooking process. Place in the oven for approximately 2 hours.

Meanwhile, to make the pumpkin purée, add the oil to the small pot and sweat the onion and squash along with the ginger over medium heat. Pour in the water and simmer for 30 minutes, until tender. Drain and purée the squash in the blender, then season to taste.

When the beef is ready, remove it from the cooking liquid. Transfer the liquid to the large pot, add the remaining aromatics, and reduce the sauce as quickly as possible. Meanwhile, make the cucumber salad by combining the cucumber ribbons with the rest of the ingredients, tossing gently.

When the sauce has reduced and thickened, place a portion of beef on each plate, pour over some sauce, top with salad, and spoon some of the squash purée either side. Garnish with sliced radish and fresh dill, if desired.

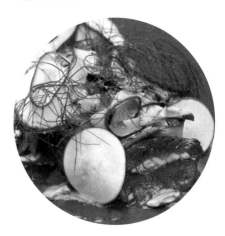

Pork schnitzel with fried egg, asparagus & tartar sauce

A classic dish that has haunted too many restaurant menus for too long, but has an undeniable appeal. You can easily substitute the pork for chicken, and you can use an alternative crumb to "bread" the meat. I find using ground almonds gives a lovely texture to the crust.

Serves   4
Prep time   20 minutes
Cooking time   20 minutes
Carb count   6.3 g per serving

EQUIPMENT

2 large shallow bowls, chopping board, knives, frying pan, baking sheet, pot of boiling salted water

INGREDIENTS

Schnitzel

1-2 eggs, beaten (depends on how much pork you are breading)
100 g (1 cup) ground almonds
600 g (1⅓ lb) pork tenderloin
salt and pepper to taste
15 g (1 Tbsp) butter

Accompaniments

4-8 eggs (1-2 per person)
1-2 Tbsp butter
300 g (3 cups) asparagus (or green beans, depending on season)
60 ml (¼ cup) Tartar Sauce (page 132)

METHOD

Preheat the oven to 350°F. Place the beaten egg and ground almonds in separate large, shallow bowls. Holding the knife parallel to the cutting board, slice horizontally through the pork tenderloin, stopping ⅜ inch before you slice right through. Unfold the pork and lightly bat with a heavy implement (a meat hammer is perfect, but a rolling pin or a heavy saucepan will also do the trick). Flatten to a thickness of about ¼ inch.

Cut the flattened pork into 4 equal serving pieces. Dip each piece into the beaten egg and then place it on a plate while you dip the rest. Season with salt and pepper. Next, coat the meat in the ground almonds and place on another plate. Repeat until all the meat is completely coated. Panfry the schnitzel in the butter until golden on each side, then transfer it to the baking sheet and place in the oven to finish cooking for 6-8 minutes.

Fry the eggs in the butter and boil the asparagus for 2 minutes, until tender. Serve the schnitzel with the asparagus and eggs, and spoon over some tartar sauce - or whatever sauce you like. Tomato Salsa (page 133) also works well here, but the tartar is my favorite.

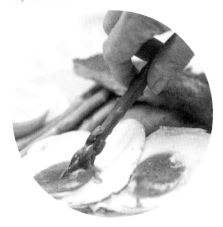

Where are my noodles?

Sometimes it's nice to accompany dishes with the thing they go hand in hand with. Bangers and mash, curry and rice, bread and everything – the list is endless. The recipes that follow are designed to fill that gap in your meal planning, with the added bonus of not pushing you past the threshold of prediabetes. Plus, they are way more nutritious than filler foods such as year-old pasta.

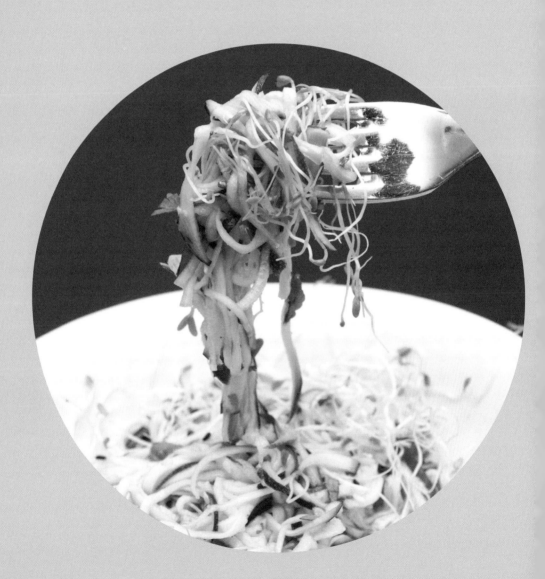

Zucchini noodles

The perfect pasta replacement.

Serves   2
Prep time   10 minutes
Cooking time   3 minutes
Carb count   2.3 g per serving

EQUIPMENT
Mandolin or slicer side of a grater (optional), chopping board, knife, frying pan

INGREDIENTS
2-3 zucchini
salt and pepper to taste
5 ml (1 tsp) olive oil

METHOD
Slice the zucchini into strips about ¹⁄₁₆ inch thick and then cut into long threads. Season with salt and pepper and lightly sauté with the olive oil for 1 minute. You can let them cool, store in the fridge, and then boil them straight from the fridge for 2 minutes to accompany a pasta sauce, or cook them as you need them to accompany your main meal.

Instead of all that chopping, you could also use a julienne peeler. Alternatively, use a simple peeler to get a flat, ribbon-style "pappardelle" shape. Cook as above.

Creamy mash

Low carb, tasty and so easy.

Serves   3-4
Prep time   10 minutes
Cooking time   30 minutes
Carb count   5 g per serving (using celery root)

EQUIPMENT
Chopping board, knives, large pot of boiling water, colander, food processor or blender or masher

INGREDIENTS
1 medium head cauliflower, cut into florets
1 celery root, peeled and cut into 1-inch cubes
    (optional)
125 ml (½ cup) cream
50 g (¼ cup) butter
salt and pepper to taste

METHOD
Having peeled, prepped, and cut the veggies, add them to the pot with the rest of the ingredients and simmer for 20-30 minutes. Drain in the colander, reserving the liquid as it passes through. Combine the vegetables, reserved liquid, and seasoning in a food processor (or whatever you are using). Purée the vegetables to your preferred consistency, adjusting the thickness to your liking with the reserved liquid. Feel free to play around by adding herbs, mustard, or cheese to the mash. For example, adding an egg yolk gives a great golden, crusty topping to Fish Pie (page 138).

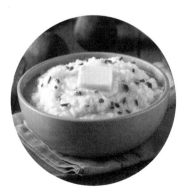

Cauliflower rice

A classic low-carb recipe that is quick and versatile.

Serves   2-3
Prep time   10 minutes
Cooking time   10 minutes
Carb count   2.7 g (rice); 5.1 g (pilau)
                per serving

EQUIPMENT
Chopping board, knife, food processor,
pot with a lid

INGREDIENTS
½ medium head cauliflower, cut into florets
20 g (1½ Tbsp) butter
60 ml (¼ cup) water
salt and pepper to taste

METHOD
Pulse the raw cauliflower in a food processor
until it resembles small grains of rice. Melt the
butter in the pot and sauté the cauliflower for
1 minute. Add in the water and the salt and
pepper, put on the lid, and cook over low heat
for 6-8 minutes. The "rice" is nicer if it retains
a little bite, similar to conventional rice.

Pilau variation

INGREDIENTS
1 onion, diced
1 clove garlic, crushed
3 g (½ tsp) crushed ginger
20 g (1½ Tbsp) butter or coconut oil
salt and pepper to taste
3 g (½ tsp) garam masala
3 g (½ tsp) ground coriander
3 g (½ tsp) turmeric
cauliflower rice (as cooked above)

METHOD
Sweat the onion, garlic, and ginger in the butter or
oil over medium heat. Add in the salt, pepper, and
spices and cook out the rawness for 1 minute. Stir in
the cauliflower rice.

Oven fries

You simply cannot go without fries!

Serves   2
Prep time   5 minutes
Cooking time   30 minutes
Carb count   9.2 g per serving

EQUIPMENT
Chopping board, knives, baking sheet lined with
grease-proof paper, mixing bowl

INGREDIENTS
1 celery root
1 parsnip
60 ml (¼ cup) olive oil
salt and pepper to taste
a few sprigs rosemary (optional)
a few cloves garlic, unpeeled (optional)

METHOD
Preheat the oven to 350°F. Peel the celery root by
removing the outer skin as you would that of an
orange, and peel the parsnip as you would a carrot.
Cut the celery root into fries as thick or thin as you
like. Remove the root from the parsnip and cut it
into similar-sized pieces. Add the olive oil and salt
and pepper to a bowl along with the veggies and
toss together. Add the rosemary and garlic (if using)
and transfer to the lined baking sheet. Bake for 25-
30 minutes, or longer if necessary.

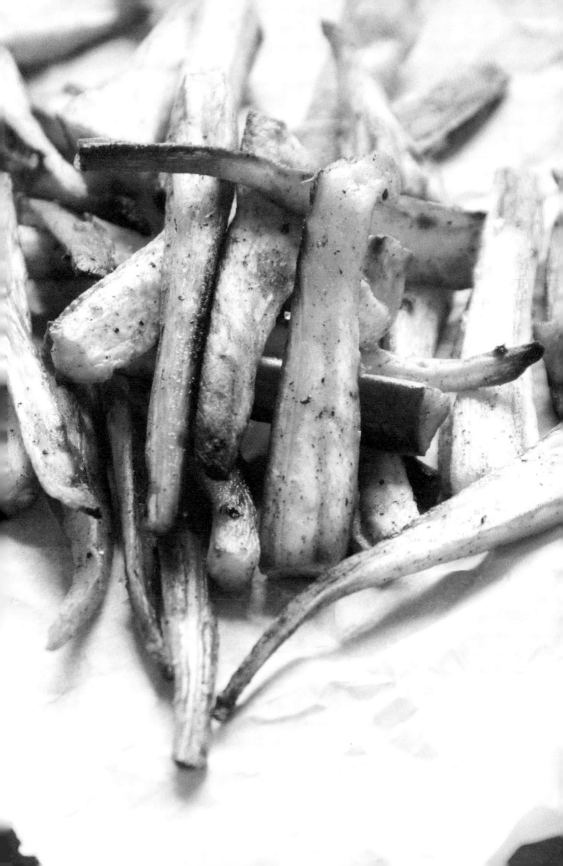

Low-carb bread

Soft and delicious, this "bread" deserves to be made and eaten.

Baking the mix in a loaf pan will result in a sliceable loaf. Muffin or cupcake pans make individual buns, or you can simply roll the mix into balls and bake on a baking sheet. Every cuisine has a way to wrap or contain food, even LCHF – the difference being that ours is very nutritious and satiating. This recipe uses a small amount of psyllium husks, which help to take up the water and hold it in the bread. You can find psyllium husks at the supermarket and also any local health-food shop. This mix will make a small- to medium-sized loaf, about 12 slices.

Makes	1 loaf or 6 buns or muffins
Prep time	15 minutes
Cooking time	25 minutes
Carb count	3.3 g (2 slices or 1 bun or muffin)

EQUIPMENT

Parchment paper (optional), muffin pan, loaf pan or baking sheet, mixing bowl, bowl scraper

INGREDIENTS

oil or butter for greasing sheet (optional)
150 g (1½ cups) almond flour (or ground almonds)
45 g (8 Tbsp) psyllium-husk powder
10 g (2 tsp) baking powder
5 g (1 tsp) salt
60 ml (¼ cup) extra-virgin olive oil (or melted butter)
4 eggs, beaten
100 g (½ cup) sour cream

METHOD

Preheat the oven to 325°F. Grease your muffin pan or loaf pan, or line whatever you will be using with parchment paper.

Combine all of the bread ingredients in the bowl and leave to stand for up to 10 minutes; the psyllium husks will take up a lot of the moisture and hold it in the mix. Once the mix is less sticky, shape the dough into balls on the lined baking sheet, or place the mixture into the greased muffin pan or loaf pan. Bake in the oven for 25 minutes (loaf) or 12 minutes (muffins or buns). To check that they're done, poke a skewer into the middle; it should come out dry.

VARIATION

- Make it a multiseed loaf by including up to 100 g (3½ oz) of your favorite seeds in whatever ratio suits. Poppy seeds, flaxseed, sesame seeds, pumpkin seeds, and sunflower seeds are all excellent options.

- The recipe can be made dairy-free by omitting the sour cream, doubling the extra-virgin olive oil to 120 ml (½ cup), and including 35 ml (2½ Tbsp) water.

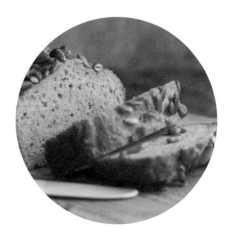

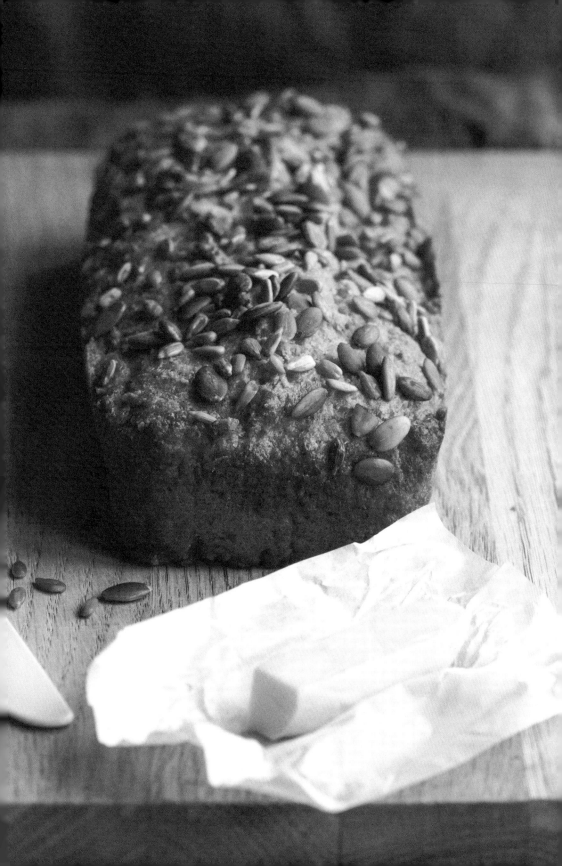

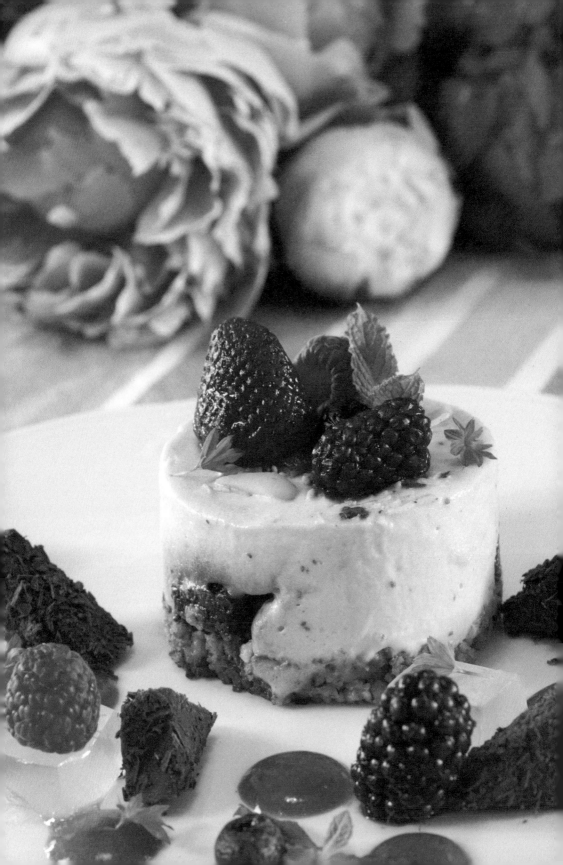

Dessert

I have to confess that, either out of habit or because of my training as a chef, there are times when I like to round off a meal with something delicious and decadent. These dessert recipes demonstrate how we can maintain our LCHF lifestyle while enjoying a little treat along the way. Continuing our emphasis on nutrient-dense ingredients, these recipes use whole foods to create desserts and small treats that will keep you on track while you indulge a little.

Coconut balls

Joyful little mouthfuls – just don't let them lead you to ruin!

Makes   16 balls
Prep time   20 minutes
Setting time   1 hour
Carb count   2.6 g (1 ball)

EQUIPMENT

Knife, chopping board, pot, whisk, baking sheet

INGREDIENTS

150 g (5 oz) dark chocolate (85% cocoa)
60 ml (¼ cup) cream
50 g (½ cup) shredded/desiccated coconut
15 g (1 Tbsp) coconut oil

For rolling

30 g (¼ cup) slivered almonds
30 g (⅓ cup) shredded coconut

METHOD

Preheat the oven to 325°F. With a large kitchen knife, cut the chocolate into small pieces. Bring the cream to a boil, add the chocolate, and whisk. Next, add the shredded coconut and coconut oil and stir to an even mix. Place in the fridge for an hour to set.

Meanwhile, toast the almonds on a baking sheet in the oven for 4 minutes, then shake or stir them to ensure even cooking, and toast in the oven for a further 3-4 minutes. The almonds should be a light golden brown. Tip them onto a plate to cool.

Roll the chocolate mix into 16 balls and coat in the slivered almonds and shredded coconut. Transfer the balls to an airtight container; they will keep in the fridge for 1-2 weeks.

Chocolate brittle peanut butter creamy delight

This recipe is not clever, it's not fancy, but it is tasty and you can make it in about ten minutes.

Serves   5-6
Prep time   10 minutes
Setting time   20 minutes
Carb count   6.3 g per serving

EQUIPMENT

Pot of hot water, heatproof bowl, food processor or pestle and mortar, mixing bowl, whisk, baking sheet lined with parchment paper

INGREDIENTS

Chocolate brittle

100 g (3½ oz) dark chocolate (85% cocoa)
100 g (½ cup) Grain-Free Granola (page 100)

Peanut-butter cream

60 g (¼ cup) unsweetened peanut butter
125 ml (½ cup) cream, lightly whipped
a few drops of stevia (or xylitol), to taste

METHOD

Melt the chocolate in the heatproof bowl set over the pot of hot water, until smooth. Pulse the grain-free granola in the food processor, then pour it into the chocolate. Spread this mix over the lined baking sheet and cool in the fridge to form the brittle (about 20 minutes). Meanwhile, whisk together the peanut butter and cream, and season with stevia or xylitol. Break the brittle into shards and serve alongside the peanut-butter cream.

Berry & saffron chocolate truffles

Intensely enjoyable after-dinner bites that you can
make well in advance and then pull out as required.

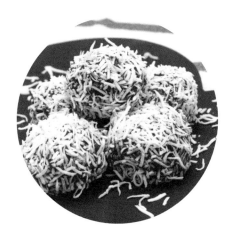

Makes	10
Prep time	20 minutes
Setting time	1 hour
Carb count	4.1 g per truffle

EQUIPMENT

Pot, blender or a mixing bowl and whisk,
small shallow container, jug of hot water,
knife, mixing bowl

INGREDIENTS

60 ml (¼ cup) cream
60 ml (¼ cup) berry purée (see page 162)
pinch of saffron (optional)
150 g (5 oz) dark chocolate (85% cocoa), chopped
7 g (1 Tbsp) cocoa powder
10 fresh raspberries

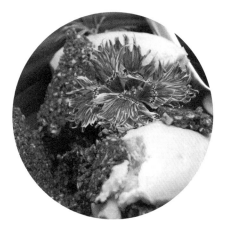

METHOD

Bring the cream, berry purée, and saffron (if using)
to a boil in the pot. Put the chocolate in the blender
(or the mixing bowl) and pour over the very hot
cream mix. Blend or whisk to a smooth, thick
ganache. The blender is preferred because it creates
a more emulsified ganache, but this recipe doesn't
need to be too particular. Transfer to the shallow
container and allow to set in the fridge for 1 hour.

Once set, cut into squares, using some hot water
on your knife for a nice clean cut. Place the cocoa
in the mixing bowl and add the squares. Rotate the
bowl to coat the squares, then transfer them to an
airtight container. They will keep in the fridge for
up to 2 weeks, and up to 3 months in the freezer.
Defrost in the fridge if frozen, and top with a fresh
raspberry before serving.

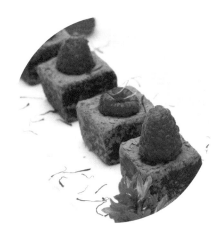

Rocky road slice

Yes, this involves gelatin, but don't be scared – it's just another culinary frontier to add to your ever-growing skill set. Cut into small cubes, this makes a great low-carb treat. The different textures are the secret to these little bites.

Makes	about 20 pieces
Prep time	20 minutes
Setting time	1½ hours
Carb count	3.3 g (1 piece)

EQUIPMENT

Stand blender or hand blender, sieve, mixing bowls, scales, 2 pots, small plastic container, knife, chopping board, ovenproof dish, large plate, straight-sided shallow baking pan

INGREDIENTS

Berry purée jelly
200 g (2 cups) mixed frozen berries
1 sheet gelatin

15 g (2 Tbsp) hazelnuts
15 g (2 Tbsp) almonds
15 g (2 Tbsp) macadamias
15 g (3 Tbsp) shelled pistachios
50 g (3-4) Coconut Balls (page 160)
180 g (6 oz) dark chocolate (85% cocoa)
75 ml (⅓ cup) cream
shredded/desiccated coconut, to garnish

METHOD

Make the berry purée by blitzing the frozen berries for 1 minute, until loose and smooth. Pass through a sieve and weigh out 100 g (5 Tbsp) of the purée, reserving the rest for adding to yogurt or similar – it will last 5 days in the fridge.

Soften the gelatin in cold water, and gently heat the berry purée. When the gelatin is soft, remove it from the water and squeeze out the excess liquid. Add the gelatin to the warmed purée and stir until dissolved. Pour the liquid jelly into the plastic container and set in the fridge – after 30 minutes, it will be set enough to cut into small cubes.

Preheat the oven to 350°F. Toast the nuts in the ovenproof dish for 5 minutes, stir, and then toast for 2-3 minutes longer to cook evenly. Transfer the nuts to the large plate and set to one side to cool.

Break the coconut balls up into chunks. With a large kitchen knife, finely chop 150 g (5 oz) of the chocolate and place in a mixing bowl. Chop the remaining chocolate into chunks and set aside. Heat the cream until close to a boil, then whisk it through the finely chopped chocolate to form a ganache.

Assemble the slice by pouring the ganache into the baking pan, then arrange all the other ingredients on the soft ganache, pressing them in a little – the jelly cubes, the toasted nuts, the dark chocolate chunks, and the coconut balls broken up into smaller chunks. Chill for 1 hour, then cut into pieces and keep in an airtight container in the fridge. Sprinkle some coconut over the slice before serving.

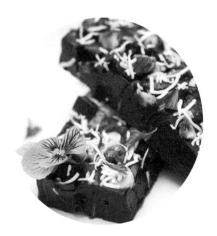

Coconut panna cotta with pineapple, mango & chili mint salsa

A perfect light and clean dessert, although you'll need to prepare it in advance due to the three-hour setting time. Served with a little bit of the salsa, it makes for a low-carb tropical hit.

Serves	4
Prep time	15 minutes
Cooking time	5 minutes
Setting time	3 hours
Carb count	10.2 g per serving

EQUIPMENT

Chopping board, knives, pot, ring molds or glasses, bowl of hot water

INGREDIENTS

Panna cotta

3½ sheets gelatin
250 ml (1 cup) cream
375 ml (1½ cups) coconut milk
50 g (¼ cup) young coconut flesh, diced (optional)
stevia to taste

Salsa

½–1 chili, de-seeded and finely diced
¼ pineapple, peeled and diced small
½ mango, peeled and diced small
15 g (1 Tbsp) chopped fresh mint
zest and juice of 1 lime

METHOD

Soften the gelatin in cold water, and gently heat the cream and coconut milk. When the gelatin is soft, squeeze out the excess water and add it to the hot cream mix, stirring until dissolved. Mix in the coconut flesh (if using) and the stevia. Set the mix in the ring molds or glasses in the fridge.

Prepare all the salsa ingredients and marinate with the lime zest and juice for as long as the panna cotta takes to set, about 3 hours. De-mold the panna cottas by dipping the molds or glasses in hot water and turning out, and spoon over some of the salsa to serve.

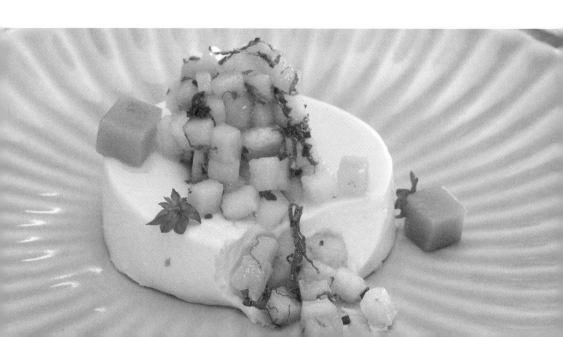

Berry cheesecake

When my wife, Hailey, said, "We need an LCHF cheesecake on the menu!," the challenge was set.
Luckily, my first attempt made the grade. If fresh berries aren't in season, just defrost frozen ones.

Serves	6
Prep time	40 minutes
Setting time	1 hour
Carb count	24 g (with the extras);
	7.9 g (without) per serving

EQUIPMENT

Food processor, sieve, mixing bowls, whisk, cutting boards, knives, heatproof bowl, pot of hot water, 6 ring molds (or 1 cake pan with its removable base removed and placed directly on a cutting board)

INGREDIENTS

Filling

30 g (¼ cup) raspberries
30 g (4 medium) strawberries
30 g (¼ cup) blueberries
30 g (¼ cup) blackberries
250 ml (1 cup) cream
zest of 1 lemon
3-4 drops stevia (optional)
seeds scraped from ½ vanilla pod (or 2-3 drops
    of extract)
250 g (1 cup) mascarpone

Base

50 g (2 oz) dark chocolate (85% cocoa), chopped,
plus 50 g (2 oz) for shaving
100 g (½ cup) Grain-Free Granola (page 100)
50 g (¼ cup) butter, melted
1 Tbsp (2-3 small) raspberries
1 Tbsp (2-3 small) strawberries

Extras to serve (per person)

3 berries
2 small Berry & Saffron Chocolate Truffles
    (page 161; optional)
2 small cubes Prosecco Jelly (page 166; optional)

METHOD

To make the berry filling, blitz the berries in the food processor for 30 seconds until puréed, and strain through the sieve. Lightly whip the cream until it is almost, but not quite, as thick as the mascarpone. Fold the cream together with the lemon zest, stevia, vanilla, and mascarpone. Ripple through about one-third of the berry filling, saving the rest for when you plate up.

Melt the chopped chocolate for the base in the heatproof bowl set over the pot of hot water, off the heat. Pulse the grain-free granola in the food processor until it is small and grainy. Pour in the chocolate and the melted butter and mix until combined. Line the base of the molds or pan with the granola mix and compress nicely. Place 3 berries in each individual mold, or make a ring of berries around the outside of the cake pan. Spoon in the filling mix and smooth over with a knife heated in hot water. Shave some chocolate over the top and allow to set in the fridge for 1 hour. De-mold each cheesecake by running your knife around the edge and lifting the ring away. Serve on plates with some of the reserved sauce and a few extra berries, plus the optional extras if desired.

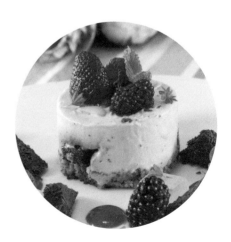

Decadent chocolate mousse with orange ice cream

If you don't have an ice cream maker, you can set the mix in the freezer and whisk the ice crystals from time to time as it sets. For the ultimate shortcut version, simply zest the orange into some whipped cream sweetened with stevia, and serve straight from the fridge.

Serves	6–8
Prep time	25 minutes
Cooking time	5 minutes
Setting time	up to 3 hours
Carb count	2.5 g per serving

EQUIPMENT

Blender, ice cream maker or freezer container, whisk, stand mixer with whisk attachment, heatproof bowl, mixing bowl, pot of hot water, glasses or molds

INGREDIENTS

Ice cream

6 eggs
2 egg yolks
60 ml (¼ cup) cream
zest of 1 orange
15 ml (1 Tbsp) fresh orange juice
125 g (½ cup) butter
125 g (½ cup) coconut oil
8–10 drops stevia

Mousse

5 egg yolks
75 g (2½ oz) dark chocolate (85% cocoa),
    broken up into small pieces
75 ml (⅓ cup) cream
few drops of stevia to taste
zest of ½ orange
small pinch of sea salt

fresh fruit for garnish (optional)

METHOD

Blitz the ice cream ingredients in the blender for 3 minutes. As the friction against the blades continues, the butter and coconut oil will melt and emulsify with the eggs. Pour the mixture into an ice cream maker or a container for the freezer. Churn, or freeze and stir as necessary, and set for 2 hours.

To make the mousse, start to whisk the egg yolks in the stand mixer. Meanwhile, sit the chocolate in the heatproof bowl set over the pot of hot water, off the heat, to gently melt. Begin to lightly whisk the cream in a separate mixing bowl. When the chocolate has melted, place all the bowls next to one another. The egg should have doubled in volume from the mixing. Fold the chocolate into the egg mix, then fold in the cream, stevia, orange zest, and sea salt. Pour the mixture into glasses or molds and set in the fridge for approximately 1 hour.

Serve the mousse with the ice cream and garnish with fresh fruit, if desired. I sometimes serve this dish in a dark-chocolate case (see below)!

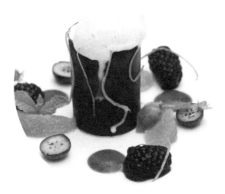

Summer berries & prosecco jelly

This prosecco jelly makes a beautiful flavor point for serving with strawberries and cream.

Serves 12
Prep time 15 minutes
Setting time 5 hours or overnight
Carb count 2.6 g per serving, including extras

EQUIPMENT
Pot, loaf pan, or a plastic container lined with plastic wrap, chopping board, knife, whisk, mixing bowls

INGREDIENTS
5 sheets gelatin
200 g (1 cup) berry purée (see page 162)
500 ml (⅔ bottle/2 cups) prosecco
50 g (½ cup) fresh raspberries
50 g (½ cup) fresh strawberries
50 g (½ cup) fresh blackberries
50 g (⅓ cup) fresh blueberries

Extras to serve (optional)
15 g (7-8) mint leaves
extra berries
heavy cream

METHOD
Soften the sheets of gelatin in cold water. Heat the berry purée; when the gelatin is soft, squeeze out the excess water and stir it into the hot purée until dissolved. Cool for 30 minutes, until fairly cold to the touch (use the fridge if necessary, but try not to let the jelly set). Add in the prosecco and then pour the prosecco jelly to halfway up the loaf pan, reserving some jelly for later. Set in the fridge for 1½ hours, until fairly set.

Remove the pan from the fridge, push some berries into the jelly, and leave the rest on the surface. Pour over the rest of the prosecco jelly and return the pan to the fridge for 3 more hours or overnight. Turn the jelly out and cut into slices. Serve on its own or with mint, extra berries, and heavy cream.

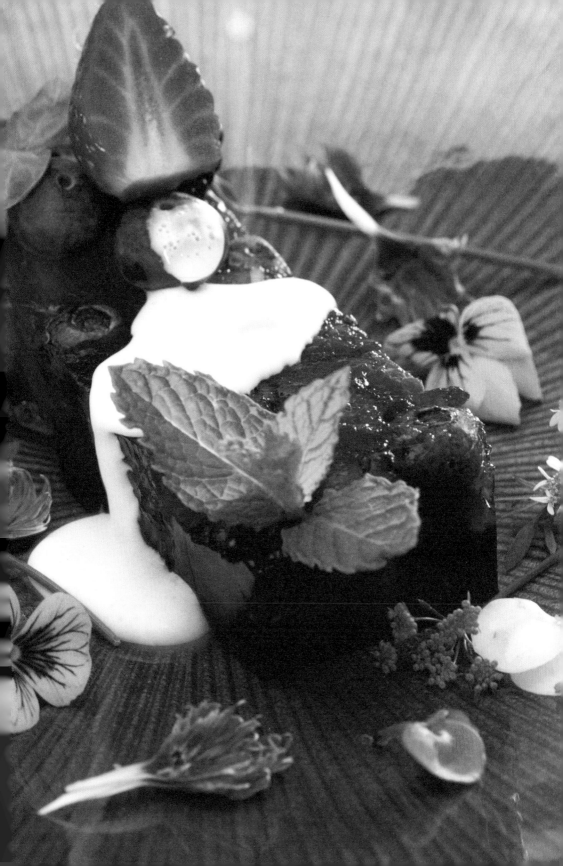

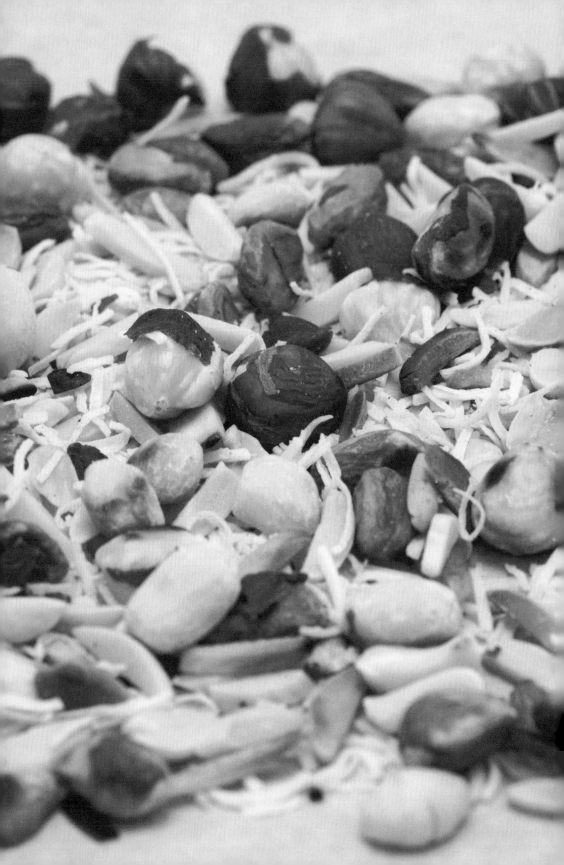

Nibbles

Creating nibbles for visitors is a great way to spend more time socializing and less time slaving in the kitchen. Having a few good nibble recipes you can whip up quickly also saves you from being stranded at parties with nothing to eat – plan ahead and turn up armed with LCHF-suitable snacks. These are just a few ideas to inspire you, from the standard chips and dips to more adventurous savory nibbles.

Chips & dips

This is a whole new take on an old favorite. Packed with a nutritious punch rather than preservatives.

Serves	6-8
Prep time	20 minutes
Cooking time	30 minutes
Carb count	7.2 g per serving

EQUIPMENT
Mandolin or slicer, chopping boards, knives, 2 baking trays, wire cooling rack, mixing bowl

INGREDIENTS
200 g (7 oz) celery root (or parsnip), peeled and sliced thinly
15 ml (1 Tbsp) olive oil
(2 medium) carrots, peeled and sliced thinly
250 g (8 oz; 4 cups) kale, picked and washed
100 g (1 scant cup) grated Parmesan
15 ml (1 Tbsp) tamari (gluten-free soy sauce)
cracked pepper to taste
60 ml (¼ cup) Mayonnaise (page 132)
60 ml (¼ cup) Guacamole (page 133)
60 ml (¼ cup) sour cream

METHOD
Preheat the oven to 325°F. The celery root takes the long-est to cook (30 minutes), so place it on a baking sheet first and drizzle over some olive oil. Put the sheet in the oven, and after 20 minutes add the carrots on the other sheet with the kale. After a further 10 minutes, remove the celery root chips and transfer to the wire rack to cool. Put the grated Parmesan on the just-used sheet and bake for 6-8 minutes – it will melt and make a cheesy sheet. When the vegetables and Parmesan come out of the oven, transfer the vegetables to the cooling rack to get crispy. Crack the Parmesan sheet into small crisps, and season the vegetable chips with some tamari and cracked pepper. Serve with the dips and bask in your guests' total admiration.

Veggies (crudités) & dips

A simpler version of the Chips & Dips recipe, but still a winner.

Serves	6
Prep time	15 minutes
Carb count	4.4 g per serving

EQUIPMENT
Chopping board, knives

INGREDIENTS
1 carrot, peeled
3 ribs celery, washed
1 bell pepper
½ English cucumber
100 g (1 cup) cherry tomatoes
50 g (½ cup) walnuts
60 ml (¼ cup) Guacamole (page 133)
60 ml (¼ cup) Tomato Salsa (page 133)
60 ml (¼ cup) sour cream
30 ml (2 Tbsp) Vinaigrette (page 131)

METHOD
Cut the carrot, celery, and bell pepper into little sticks. Cut the cucumber in half lengthwise and scoop out the seeds with a spoon. Then cut into small sticks. Assemble the vegetables and nuts on a plate and serve with the dips.

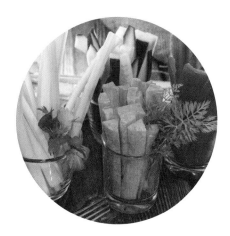

Caesar & smoked salmon Waldorf micro salads

Romaine lettuce leaves make great serving dishes and are a fun way to serve these classic salads. Keep a range of toasted nuts in the pantry – they are very versatile and can add texture to your food, like in the Waldorf salad here.

Makes	Enough for 12 canapé-style portions
Prep time	30 minutes
Carb count	0.2 g (Caesar); 0.5 g (Waldorf) per portion

EQUIPMENT
Chopping boards, knives

INGREDIENTS
Caesar salad
2 boiled eggs (see page 96 for instructions)
30 ml (2 Tbsp) Caesar Dressing (page 130)
1 slice cooked bacon, crumbled, plus extra for garnish (optional)
1 head romaine lettuce, shredded
salt and pepper to taste
2-3 anchovies

Waldorf salad
12 toasted walnuts (see page 100 for instructions)
15 g (1 Tbsp) cream cheese
15 g (1 Tbsp) sliced chives
15 g (2½ Tbsp) diced red onion
50 g (2 oz) smoked salmon
15 g (2½ Tbsp) diced celery
salt and pepper to taste

To serve
12 small romaine lettuce leaves

METHOD
For the Caesar: peel and slice the eggs and combine with the dressing, bacon, and shredded lettuce. Season the mix, spoon it into 6 of the lettuce leaves and garnish with a piece of anchovy or sliver of bacon.

For the Waldorf: chop the walnuts roughly and mix with the cream cheese, chives, and most of the red onion. Spoon the mix into the other 6 lettuce leaves. Drape pieces of salmon on top, and garnish with the celery and the remaining red onion. Season to taste.

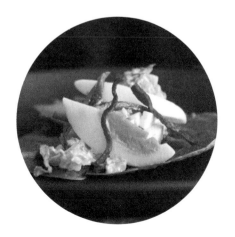 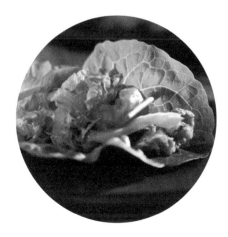

Prosciutto-wrapped asparagus

A simple but crowd-pleasing nibble to start off an evening. These can be prepared a day in advance, although they take no time to make.

Makes	4-6 portions
Prep time	10 minutes
Carb count	0.8 g (per wrapped spear)

EQUIPMENT

Chopping board, knife, pot of boiling water, bowl of cold water

INGREDIENTS

12 spears asparagus
60 g (2 oz; 12 small slices) prosciutto

METHOD

Trim the ends of the asparagus as long or short as you like – just ensure that you have removed the woody base if you leave them long. Blanch the asparagus in the boiling water for 2-3 minutes, depending on the thickness of the stems. Cool the asparagus in the cold water, then wrap the bases in the prosciutto.

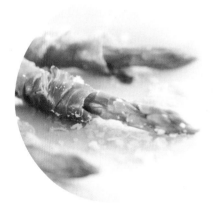

Cheese & crackers

A cheese board is a great way to wind down a meal or to continue an evening. The recipe for these crackers is very versatile and I am really happy with their texture and shortness. It makes twelve crackers, depending on how big you cut them. Don't be scared to reroll the cuttings, as without the gluten they won't become tough with rerolling.

Prep time	25 minutes
Cooking time	30 minutes
Carb count	2.4 g (2 crackers, 1 tsp jam, cheese wedge, 8-10 nuts)

EQUIPMENT

Food processor, plastic wrap, rolling pin, cookie cutter, baking sheet lined with parchment paper, chopping board, knife, frying pan, mixing bowl

INGREDIENTS

Almond crackers

30 g (2 Tbsp) butter, cold from the fridge
175 g (1¾ cup) ground almonds
½ tsp salt
5 g (1 tsp) chopped fresh rosemary
1 egg

Onion jam

15 ml (1 Tbsp) olive oil
2 onions, finely sliced
75 ml (⅓ cup) red wine
1 star anise
½ stick cinnamon
salt and pepper to taste

Cheese & nuts

30 g (1 oz) cheddar
30 g (1 oz) blue cheese
30 g (1 oz) soft brie-style cheese
10 g (4-5) toasted almonds (see page 100 for instructions)
10 g (8-10) toasted pistachios (see page 100 for instructions)

METHOD

In the food processor, blend all the ingredients for the crackers except the egg. When the mixture resembles crumbs, add the egg and stop blending as it begins to clump. Spread some plastic wrap out on your work surface and then scoop the contents of the food processor onto the plastic wrap. Spread a second sheet of plastic wrap over the mixture so that the cracker mixture is sandwiched between the two layers of wrap. You can use the plastic wrap roll as a rolling pin (or use an actual rolling pin). Roll the cracker mixture until it is thin, like a cracker, approximately 1/16 inch thick. Keeping it wrapped, carefully transfer the sheet of cracker mix to the fridge to rest for 30 minutes.

Preheat the oven to 325°F. When the mix has rested, cut the crackers out using a cookie cutter or knife. Transfer the raw crackers to the lined baking sheet and cook until golden, about 8-10 minutes.

Meanwhile, to make the jam, heat the olive oil in the frying pan and cook the onions on medium heat until beginning to color. Add the wine, spices, and seasoning, and cook covered with a lid over low heat for 15 minutes, until the onions are very soft. Remove the lid and continue to cook until the liquid has evaporated and the onions are thick and rich. Remove the onions from the heat and transfer to a bowl to cool.

Arrange the cheese and nuts on a serving plate, making sure you remove the cheese from the fridge 1 hour prior to eating to allow it to reach optimal eating temperature. Serve the onion jam and the crackers alongside the cheese and nuts.

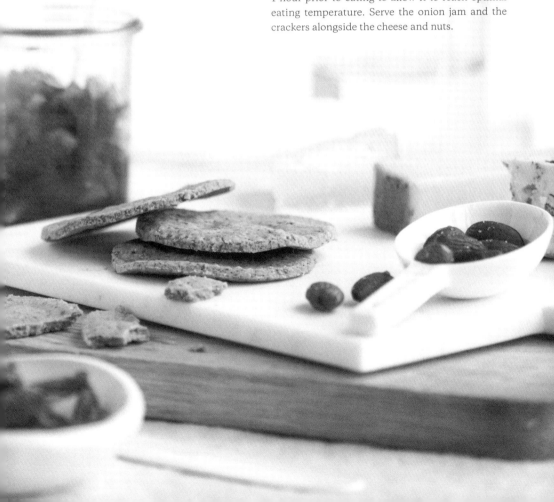

Chicken-liver pâté

This recipe is a firm favorite of mine. I love pâté, but over the years learned to associate it with brioche (that decadent, buttery French bread) and red wine–rich onion jams. My mission was to make a dish that captured the pleasure of eating pâté, but without any feeling of depriving myself of the full pâté experience. You need to make this recipe – I promise it will reward you tenfold, as it freezes well and is extremely nutritious. It's also great with steak or whisked into sauces served with meat. It lasts five days in the fridge and up to a month in the freezer. Divide the finished product up and freeze some, or better still, give it to a friend who needs to know just how good a cook you really are. Place it in the fridge for about sixteen hours to fully defrost.

Serves	12
Prep time	30 minutes
Cooking time	up to 1½ hours
Cooling time	3 hours
Carb count	2.5 g (1 Tbsp pâté, 1 Tbsp jam, 2 almond crackers)

To serve
2 Almond Crackers (page 172) per person
15 g (1 Tbsp) Onion Jam (page 172) per person
1 small beet, peeled and diced
4 sprigs parsley, chopped
a few chives, chopped

EQUIPMENT
Scales, chopping board, knife, frying pan, pot, mixing bowl, food processor, fine-mesh sieve, loaf pan, plastic wrap, spatula, tin foil, large deep oven dish, meat thermometer

INGREDIENTS
15 ml (1 Tbsp) olive oil
500 g (1 lb) chicken livers
    (duck livers are excellent, too)
600 g (1⅓ lb/2⅔ cups) butter, melted
60 g (½ cup) shallots, sliced
5 g (1 tsp) crushed garlic
5 g (1 tsp) chopped fresh thyme
zest of 1 orange
45 ml (3 Tbsp) brandy
45 ml (3 Tbsp) port
3 egg yolks
1 egg white
30 g (2 Tbsp) salt
5 g (1 tsp) ground pepper

METHOD

Preheat the oven to 275°F. Weigh out and prepare all the ingredients. Heat the frying pan over high heat and add the olive oil. Begin to fry the livers over the high heat until brown on one side. Remove from the pan and place on a plate to stop the cooking.

In the pot, use a small amount of the butter to gently sweat the shallots and the garlic over medium heat for 2 minutes. Add the thyme, orange zest, brandy, and port to the onions and garlic. Reduce the mixture over medium heat for 2 more minutes and then pour into the mixing bowl. Add the livers, onion/garlic mixture, and egg yolks and white to the food processor. Begin to blend the ingredients and then pour in the remaining melted butter in a steady stream. Pass the mixture through the sieve and then stir in the salt and pepper.

Line the loaf pan with a layer of plastic wrap - this ensures that the pâté will come out of the pan after cooking (this isn't essential - you can simply bake it directly in the pan, but you will have a paste that is spreadable from the pan instead of a sliceable, free-standing pâté). Pour the mixture into the lined pan and wrap the top of the pan with plastic wrap and foil. Half-fill the large oven dish with hot water. Place the loaf pan in the oven dish and carefully place the whole thing in the oven to cook. The time will vary from 40 minutes to an hour.

After 40 minutes, check the core temperature by probing the mixture carefully with the meat thermo-meter. The temperature should reach a minimum of 150°F - the residual heat will continue to raise the temperature, so it's important not to go too high and risk overcooking the pâté. Once the correct temperature is reached, remove the pâté from the oven, take the loaf pan out of the oven dish, and let it cool for 30 minutes. Transfer it to the fridge to fully cool for 3 hours before serving.

Serve the pâté with almond crackers and onion jam, garnishing with the beet, parsley, and chives.

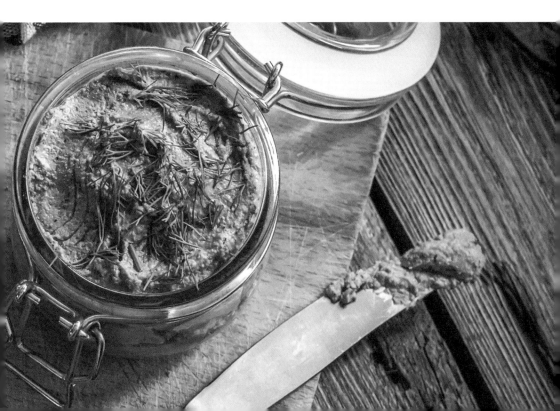

Flip the food pyramid; lose 33 pounds and feel great!

SHEREE NICHOLAS, 47, OWNER OF AN EXECUTIVE COACHING AND FACILITATION BUSINESS

New year, new me. It was the usual start to the year, with a promise to do better, especially to eat healthier. I was sluggish, had put on some weight, and wanted to re-energize.

Easy, I know how to eat. I don't have a sweet tooth, so sugar isn't an issue. All I need to be is a bit stricter on the low-fat regime. Enter my friend Katie. She tells me I've got it all wrong, in fact I was eating loads of hidden sugar – which is the real enemy – and that I needed to actually eat more fat!

Really? I think I need to do more of my own research. That research was even more confusing than enlightening. There were (and still are) so many schools of thought – Primal, Paleo, Atkins, Low Carb High Fat, Real Food. All with a slightly different take. So I decided to take the things they did agree on that are not great for us – refined sugar, processed carbohydrates, and highly processed fats – and do an experiment of n = 1 (i.e., me).

What happened?

The first thing that I noticed, within a couple of days, was the increased energy, something my family all commented on. I was having trouble sitting still (the week before, I was having trouble getting moving!) and was more productive at work. I was expecting to feel bad, but ended up feeling fantastic.

Then the weight started dropping off. The first 22 pounds vanished over 4 months, and the weight has slowly continued to disappear. A couple of visits to Dr. Caryn Zinn helped me sort through some of the mixed messages and get clear on what I wanted to focus on.

"For me, it is an ongoing experiment as I continue to learn how my body changes; both in how it looks and, much more importantly, how it feels."

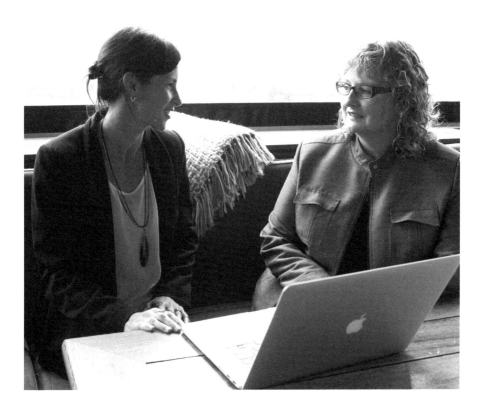

The biggest benefit and surprise to me has been the positive health impact. Last winter was the first I can recall with no sinus infection – I usually get 2 or 3 each year, often with a chest infection, and need both antibiotics and steroids to control them.

Another surprise was just how satisfied the food made me. The mid-afternoon slump was gone. Learning to tune in to what my body was telling me instead of eating because it was breakfast or lunch time was enlightening. I now don't feel the gnawing hunger I did previously. Instead of the sugar highs and lows from the processed-carb roller coaster, my energy levels are very even.

Explaining yourself

When you lose weight, people naturally want to know what you are doing. The hardest part is explaining to people that LCHF is not a diet, it is a change in perspective on what healthy eating is. The best way to describe it is that we're cutting out processed foods and eating whole foods.

There is no ingredient list because the food itself is the ingredient. For me, it is an ongoing experiment as I continue to learn how my body changes; both in how it looks and, much more importantly, how it feels. Everyone is different, so do your own experiment and see what works for you.

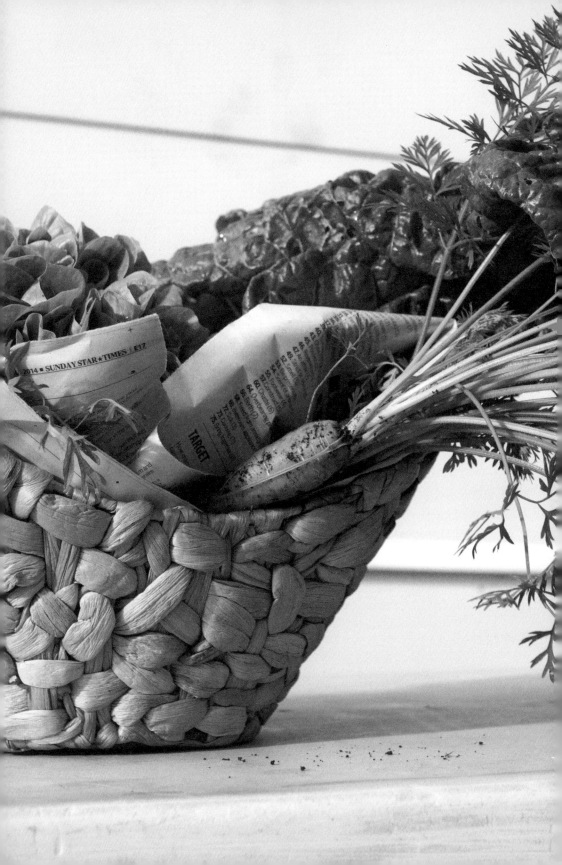

Part 3
Unlocking the real science

Hi, it's me, Grant.

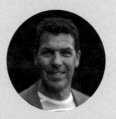

In this section, I examine the real truth about fat and look at the science behind why low-carb diets work. In doing so, I use the real-life stories of Mary, Lawrence, and Leanne to guide you through what is, at times, some pretty complicated science. That's why I'm writing this. To make it simpler to understand, and to reassure you that there is science – previously ignored, misunderstood, and sometimes even suppressed – that can help you get in shape, stay in shape, and realize your human potential.

Sure, you can go ahead, get started on LCHF, and see how it works for you. But if you want to unlock the whole truth, then it's worth considering human biology for a moment, and how food affects it. We know you want the evidence. We also know that understanding the evidence (the how and the why it works) is important for sustaining your motivation for change.

Read on for my verdict . . . the Fat Professor's verdict! By cutting through the myths and misinformation and understanding the actual science, you'll learn that:

- Eating the LCHF way proves to be the best diet for weight loss.
- Eating fat doesn't make you fat (or unhealthy).
- Saturated fat is not the big baddie you have been led to believe it is.
- All your key blood markers for cardiovascular disease improve on an LCHF diet.

Meet Mary, Lawrence & Leanne

While each of their stories is different, they have all struggled with traditional weight-loss regimes.

Mary's proof

Mary is 64 and has been overweight her whole life. She was in okay shape before her 3 children, but going through motherhood, middle age, and now into older age, she has struggled. At the end of last year, Mary was a Type 2 diabetic and on medication for diabetes and high blood pressure, plus a statin for her high cholesterol. It's not as though Mary just lost control and doesn't care about her weight. In fact, it's just the opposite. Mary cares deeply about her health and how she looks and feels. She has tried so hard. "I've listened to everything my doctor has told me over the years," says Mary. "I've tried every single type of diet that is possible. Nothing has worked. Sometimes I have lost some weight, but I always fall off the wagon and put all the weight back on again. I'm so frustrated. I'm now getting a bit older, I have diabetes, and even though I try so hard, nothing works. Why me? Why can my husband, Ron, stay so thin when he eats much less healthily than I do? I'm fat. I hate being fat. I think about it all the time."

Lawrence's proof

Lawrence is 18. He's been a fat kid, and is now a very big young man. "I've always been Big Lawrence. It's just me, the big guy, always hopeless at sports, the last one picked for games," he says. "I've hidden behind my weight problem my whole life by being the funny guy. With my mates, I'd always act that out."

When Lawrence sat in my office and I asked him if he thought much about his weight, he replied, with an unwanted tear sneaking out of the corner of his eye and sliding down his cheek, "Yeah, I do." When I asked how much, he replied, "Ninety-nine point nine percent of the time."

Lawrence came to me after he developed prediabetes and his specialist gave him a stern talking-to about his lack of willpower and how he needed to try harder to lose weight by following the low-fat food pyramid guidelines. When Lawrence said he was trying and nothing much was working, the specialist told him to try harder and to tell the truth about his exercise and nutrition habits.

Leanne's proof

Leanne had been in great shape her whole life. First she was a high-school swimmer and then she got into triathlons as a young woman. Pretty good at sports, she never worried much about her diet other than eating enough to have the energy she needed. She liked food and had a self-confessed "sweet tooth." Now Leanne is 43, with 3 active young boys aged 13, 11 and 5. She's happily married. Ever since the boys were born, however, she hasn't been able to get her weight back down. "My body just changed, and even when I tried to exercise more, I'd get a little bit in shape and then the weight would go back on again," says Leanne. "It's been my New Year's resolution to lose weight every year for the past several years, but it hasn't worked out that way. I'm still a bit overweight. I try really hard, but I love sweet stuff. I'll eat healthily for a few weeks, then everything gets too hard and I'm back eating the naughty stuff again. I'm often hungry. I'm now resigned to being like this forever – I've tried so hard, so many times."

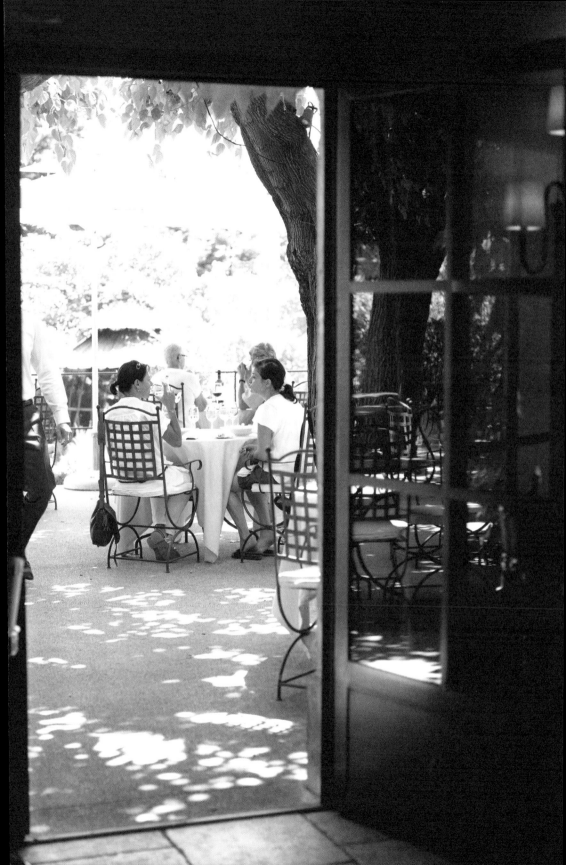

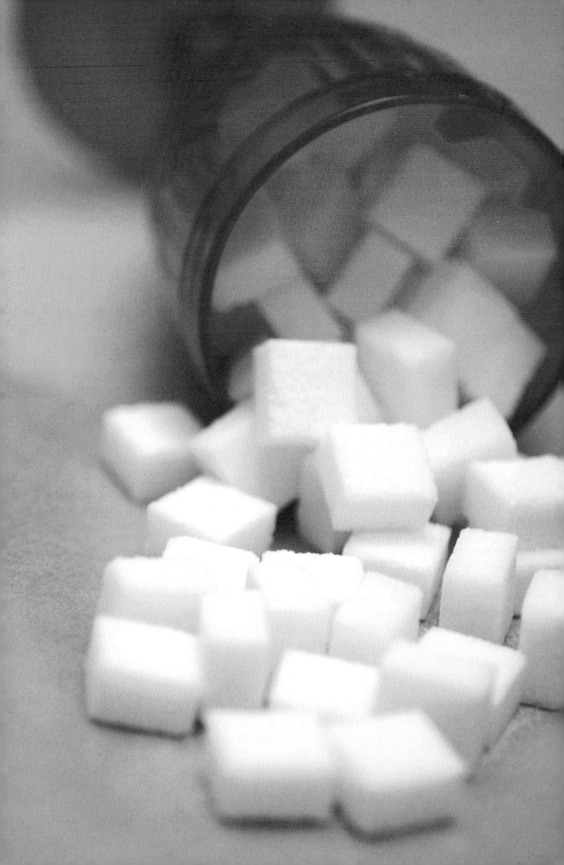

Why do we get fat?

In this section, we reveal the bad science behind popular diets and why they don't work. We begin by reviewing four of the "usual suspects" when it comes to eating and dieting. We then examine how our body works – especially how it controls hunger – and look at what Mary, Lawrence, and Leanne all have in common. We talk hormones, with the big one being insulin. It is now widely acknowledged that eating carbs raises insulin – and lots of raised insulin turns off fat burning, promotes fat storage, and makes you less active. So, the choice is simple:

• Eat whole, unprocessed foods that are low in carb, moderate in protein, and high in good-quality fat. Eating like this for life avoids insulin peaks and the eventual downward spiral into metabolic chaos that leads to weight gain.

• Or continue doing what you've always done.

The diet line-up

To understand the dynamics of LCHF, let's look at four well-known ways of eating that are in contrast to the low-carb, healthy-fat way.

The Standard American Diet (SAD)

The Standard American Diet is high carb and high fat, mostly processed and packaged food. SAD – what a great acronym, and that's how it ends: sadly . . . and badly. Your body's reaction is to raise insulin – jacked up by the carbs and sugar especially. You become "metabolically dysregulated" and store the lot.

There may even be negative synergistic effects between fats (especially saturated fats) and carbs. Remember, LCHF eating is not just a green light to increase your fat intake. If you eat fat and sugar – the most toxic carbohydrate of them all – then all bets are off as far as your health is concerned.

The low-fat diet

A low-fat diet is way better than the SAD. As the "go to" advice from governments, health promoters, doctors, and for the past 50 years, it stands as the "best way to eat" prescription that most people know and understand. It has some great things going for it. Firstly, research convincingly shows that this is a better way to eat than the SAD. Well, thank you, Captain Obvious. Secondly, it usually emphasizes whole foods, including loads of fruits and vegetables. No problems there. Thirdly, some people can get in shape and stay in shape using this approach. But here's the bad news: only some people have all the luck.

The problem with a low-fat diet is that it will be high in carbs. Unless you can cope with feeling hungry, can handle calorie deprivation, and are insulin sensitive, it won't work for you. Science has known this for a while: a 2002 Cochrane review[1] advised against low-fat diets for weight loss due to the lack of evidence that they actually work in the long term.

The Mediterranean diet

This is the low-fat diet with a bit more fat added. The Mediterranean diet generally works better than the low-fat approach, probably because the more fat you add, the less carbs you eat. But modern medicine rarely explains its success that way. They think it's the addition of better-quality food and whole grains that make it sometimes work. In reality, these higher-fat diets get part of the way there.

The high-protein diet

A high-protein diet can help people do better than the SAD and the low-fat diet. However, I caution against it – for the principal reason that as you exceed your body's requirement for daily protein, that extra protein gets turned into carbs anyway (albeit inefficiently) via a process called gluconeogenesis. Consequently, a high-protein, high-fat diet eventually resembles the SAD because you end up with higher carbs through this conversion process.

A low-fat, high-protein diet eventually resembles the low-fat diet, and isn't suitable for those who are insulin resistant. You might do slightly better because protein is satiating (filling), and that process of turning protein into carbs uses a lot of energy. Based on this, my advice is that you should only ever eat a moderate-protein diet. Our scientific detractors often tell us to stop promoting a high-protein diet. Let's just make it clear: LCHF does not mean high protein.

Our verdict

Eat a low-carb, *healthy*-fat diet (with moderate protein). This is what I'm talking about, and if you are this far into the book you'll already know most of what we are proposing. We are talking whole, actual plants and animals – foods that have a low Human Interference (HI) factor. These foods tend to be high in natural, unprocessed, "healthy" fats, low in carbohydrates, and moderate in protein. The exact amount of carbs you eat depends on your individual preferences and metabolic requirements. If you have a history of excess weight and metabolic dysregulation, then you will need to eat less carbs. If you are young and insulin sensitive, the chances are you can tolerate more carbs. That doesn't mean that insulin-sensitive people have to eat more carbs, it just means they have the option.

Imprisoned by the food pyramid

There is a saying in public health that describes the weight-loss journey. It has driven policy and practice for decades. It's "Eat less, move more." This saying describes the fundamental problem with getting too fat, not losing weight, and getting in and out of shape. To allow something to accumulate in our energy stores, the "energy in" must exceed the "energy out"; thus, conventional wisdom says that to prevent or reverse weight gain, it's crucial to eat less and move more. But why do some people get fat while others do not? Why can some people lose weight and others can't, despite being exposed to the exact same environmental conditions (the same energy in, energy out)? Because fat storage is not a simple equation of calories in and calories out – not for many people, anyway.

This is where the conventional wisdom on diet and health starts to break down. We start a blame game of gluttony and sloth. "If only you could exert your willpower to move more and eat less, then you would be in better shape." Statements like this have dogged the lives of people such as Lawrence. The obesity stigma is premised upon these psychological differences – perhaps even psychological weaknesses – between people. But there is a more nuanced, scientific explanation.

Sure, walking or biking to work, physical jobs, and most other forms of physical activity have been engineered out of our lives over recent decades. Sure, there is an abundant supply of cheap, processed food requiring no physical effort (calories expended) to catch it. But there is also a massive individual difference in how people react hormonally to food and exercise. It's that complex biological and hormonal environment that drives how we store and use up energy. It controls our hunger, our energy levels and our fat storage and use. The energy in, energy out principle completely overlooks this key fact.

We don't yet understand everything about the biology of the human body. We understand even less about nutrition. These are young and developing sciences. It's been said that half of what we know is wrong – we just have to figure out which half. I wholeheartedly agree. I'm not saying that I know everything about nutrition. The field will grow and, as with all science, good scientists will change their minds, increase their knowledge, and understand more.

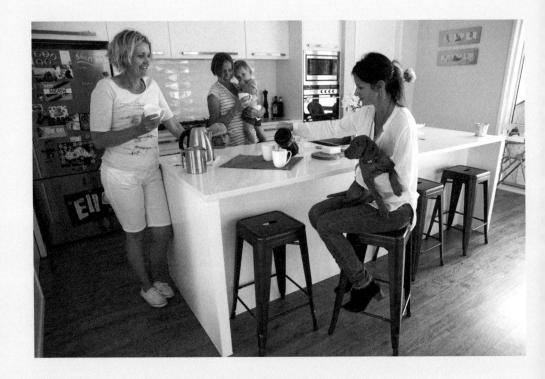

What do Mary, Lawrence & Leanne all have in common?

They have all followed conventional diet and weight-loss dogma. They all believe that if they simply had the willpower to eat less and exercise more, they would be able to get into shape. Conventional wisdom tells them that weight loss is a simple matter of calories in and calories out. Thinking this way makes it pretty obvious what to do: exercise as much as you can and eat less. But what they were not told is that the body is much more complicated than that. You see, they all have a condition - a normal human condition called insulin resistance.

Insulin is the hormone that moves blood sugar (a.k.a. blood glucose, which comes from eating carbs) around the body. It's the master hormone that controls your metabolism, driving your hunger and energy use. Mary, Lawrence, and Leanne are all trying to maintain a stable amount of sugar in their blood - about a teaspoon. When they eat more than that - say a piece of bread (equal to approximately four teaspoons of sugar) - then the body releases insulin to get rid of that extra sugar. Only in their cases, their insulin mechanism isn't working as nature designed it. They are insulin resistant, which is very common. Sugary blood is a problem for your body. It's corrosive and damages everything it touches. So your body really wants to get rid of the extra sugar.

Four things insulin does to your body

1 Eating carbs raises insulin. Insulin turns off fat burning – because you want to get rid of sugar as quickly as possible, your body will ignore all other fuel sources and just focus on the sugar.

2 Insulin tries to get sugar into cells such as the muscles and liver. That's good, but for most modern humans those cells are already full.

3 Because the insulin has nowhere else to store the carbs, it stores them as body fat.

4 Insulin disrupts the hunger and movement center in the brain. The normal feedback mechanisms that make you feel full no longer work properly, and, to make matters worse, you now feel less like being active.

That's the problem for Mary, Lawrence, and Leanne. They all tried to just eat less and exercise more. They limited their intake of fat because fat has lots of calories. They tried to live within the confines of the conventional food pyramid.

THE TROUBLE WITH THIS STRATEGY IS TWOFOLD:

1 To succeed, they'd need a serious dose of willpower to overcome the hormonally driven hunger, lack of energy, and tiredness (if they were also exercising a lot).

2 Unless they starve themselves, low-fat diets involve high carb consumption, so the problem of high insulin isn't solved.

That's why we are suggesting you flip the conventional food pyramid and eat more fat and fewer carbs (and therefore sugar). That way, you can get and stay in shape, just as Mary, Lawrence, and Leanne eventually did.

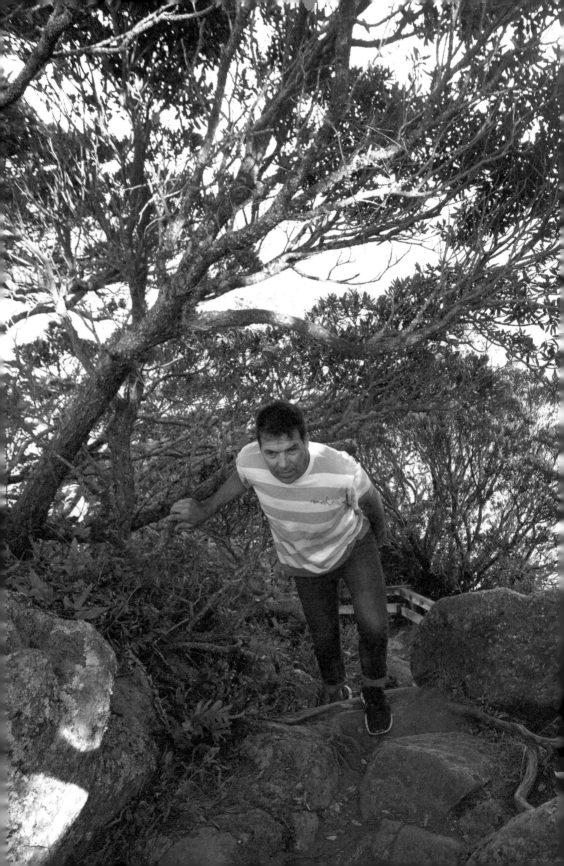

The case for being a fat burner

Okay, here we delve a little deeper into the case for fat. At times, the science does get a bit complicated. So if you're not that interested in the in-depth science, skip to the "WTF? The science in a nutshell" section on page 193.

The human fat-burning mode

There is evidence for two distinct modes of the human metabolic state. One is being "fat adapted" (also called keto-adapted). In people who are fat adapted, insulin is well controlled and the body is able to access its stores of fat as a primary source of fuel. That's worth repeating: the human body is able to primarily derive its energy from fat sources, be it dietary fat or stores of body fat. I believe that this is the normal human state, where the complex interaction of cells, hormones, enzymes, and much, much more is in balance. Fat-adapted humans homeostatically maintain a desirable body weight by self-regulating their inputs and outputs. In this state, if we overeat then we will compensate and burn it off and/or eat less; and vice versa if we undereat.

Consistent with scientific, anthropological, and clinical-practice observations, this is at least a great starting hypothesis. More good science is needed to nail all the mechanisms at work here. Putting together animal and human evidence points to this. This is why the "calorie is a calorie" dogma, which has plagued nutritional science for the past 40 years, is fundamentally wrong.

When you are "fat adapted," you burn fat easily, you have fewer cravings for refined carbs, and, most importantly, insulin is well controlled.

When they have settled into LCHF eating for a while, most people describe a switch-over in the way they access and use carbs and fat as fuel in their body. As we have discussed above, we call this being "fat adapted" or, to be more technically correct, becoming "metabolically flexible." This is the ability to switch in and out of a fat-burning state, depending on whether carbohydrate is available or not.

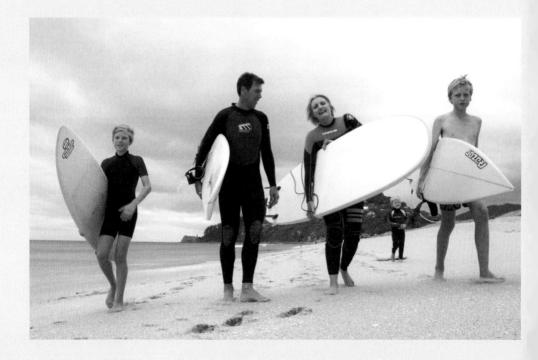

The benefits of metabolic flexibility (being "fat adapted")

Fat adaptation means burning less carbohydrate and more fat, both at rest and during moderate-intensity exercise. Less glycolysis (carbohydrate metabolism) means less oxidative stress, fewer reactive oxygen species, and fewer glycated end-products. Simply put, that's all good and means a better immune system and better health. It also means that fat is more easily burned as the primary fuel source.

Missing meals and occasional opportunistic fasting is easy to do. If you miss a meal for whatever reason, e.g., if you are served food at a function that doesn't fit with your LCHF lifestyle, as a fat-adapted individual you won't miss a beat. Fat adaptation means that you will be burning fat as a primary fuel source because insulin is kept lower across the day. Your appetite and weight-regulation system, through the hypothalamus and leptin–insulin interaction, will work as it should.[2] You are likely to feel more energetic because your brain is no longer sending signals to the rest of your nervous system to conserve energy, as it is when you are leptin resistant. It will now be easier to maintain a homeostatic weight.

Fat adaptation means saying goodbye to that terrible "glucose cliff" that most carb-dependent people fall off each day. That time of the day when the brain is saying "feed me or else" just disappears when you're on LCHF. Instead, the payback you get from eating whole foods with plenty of healthy fat is sustained energy and good mental acuity throughout the whole day.

Fat adaptation also means that you may activate more often the body's own antioxidant, gene repair, and expression system, called the histone deacetylases system. WTF? Okay, the editors have asked me to please explain this in actual English. It means that when you eat low carbs, you turn on the body's own self-defense (antioxidant) system. And believe me, that's a good thing!

Being fat adapted is like being on cruise control – no ups and no downs, just a steady state.

Metabolic dysregulation

Continually eating large amounts of carbohydrates, especially refined carbs, results in the second mode of the human metabolic state: the body becomes what I call "metabolically dysregulated." (Others use the term "metabolically deranged," but I find that a little too emotional!)

The mechanism is simplified as follows. The body produces insulin, a storage hormone, to continually deal with the large loads of dietary carbs. Insulin processes the dietary carbohydrate (and resulting sugars), but also shuts off the ability to burn fat as a fuel source. Some carbs will go into muscle cells (especially in an active individual). Some will go into the cells of the liver. The problem is that the muscle cells and liver cells are often full. This occurs because the liver has limited storage capacity and people often expend very little energy. When the liver is full, then the carbs are stored in fat cells. (That is exactly what you don't want.) This is the basic mechanism for storing fat. Insulin also drives extra fat into fat cells, too. That's why the Standard American Diet (SAD) – high fat and high carb – is particularly dangerous. So that's it. Simple. Carbohydrate consumption produces insulin. Insulin makes fat cells get bigger.

In metabolic dysregulation, the potential for a downward spiral is blatantly obvious: as you get fatter and less regulated and continue to bombard your body with large doses of dietary carbs, it's exactly like pouring fuel on a fire. You become more and more resistant to insulin, both in the muscle and the liver cells. Put simply, you need more and more insulin to get the carbs into the cells. Insulin remains permanently elevated and your cells become more resistant to their action. You are always storing fat; never burning it. A state of hyperinsulinemia (high levels of insulin in the blood) follows – even when you are not eating. You become fatter, especially around your central area. This is called visceral obesity, and it drives more inflammation and increased insulin resistance. Oh, boy!

Eventually, the beta cells in the pancreas, which produce insulin, start to fail and you can't manage your blood-sugar levels at all. That's Type 2 diabetes. And that's big trouble. Constantly high blood sugar is toxic to all parts of the body it touches, and blood sugar touches everything. That's one reason the body is so keen to get rid of carbs in the first place: high blood sugar is toxic. Your body knows it and does everything it can to get rid of it (i.e., it turns off fat-burning, and stores the carbs as fat – and insulin controls the lot).

So that is how you become metabolically dys-regulated. It is caused by lots of simple dietary carbs (i.e., sugary foods) and can be made a lot worse by a high load of carbs in general. Metabolic dysregu-lation is a pandemic. A food supply chock-full of processed carbs is to blame, but the situation is made even worse by medical recommendations to eat low-fat foods – which, sadly, more often than not are high-carb foods. It's a grim picture that explains much of our soaring national and international obesity rates.

Insulin also:

DISRUPTS LEPTIN

Leptin is a hunger hormone (the other is ghrelin). Leptin is secreted by fat cells, and sends signals to the hypothalamus in the brain that the body is not hungry. By blocking this hormone, insulin effectively disables the "not-hungry switch." When this happens, we eat – not because our body needs it, but because we are no longer receiving the signals that we are full.

DISRUPTS THE PLEASURE CENTER IN THE BRAIN

This is controlled by dopamine receptors. It is why carbs, especially sugar, are addictive in the same way that drugs such as nicotine and heroin are.

DOWN-REGULATES ACTIVITY IN THE SYMPATHETIC NERVOUS SYSTEM

This results in a reduced propensity to expend energy through both incidental and purposeful physical activity. In other words, you feel lazy and will move less.

WTF? The science in a nutshell

Metabolic dysregulation

Eating loads of carbs sends your insulin way high and leads to metabolic dysregulation, the consequences of which are:

Insulin shuts down "energy out" (energy burning).

Fat storage goes up.

Because "energy out" is synonymous with quality of life, you feel lousy.

Being metabolically well regulated is a central requirement of being the best you can be.

Being metabolically dysregulated is not your fault! Once you are on that downward escalator, it's very hard to hop off. Harder for some than others. The reason you are tired and overweight is not because you are lazy, but because you are metabolically dysregulated.

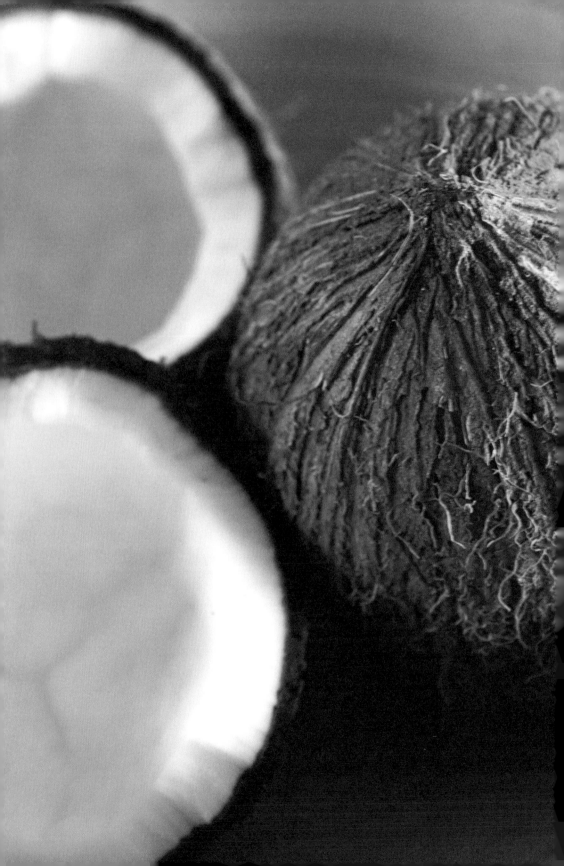

Examining the evidence for LCHF eating

In this section, Mary, Lawrence, and Leanne go LCHF. Here's what happened when they did: they got insulin under control, their bodies began to burn fat, and they experienced significant improvements in their well-being. The randomized control studies scientists run to understand the differences between people who are randomly allocated to different diets show exactly this. There are now more than 40 such studies all showing the same thing: that low-carb diets, on average, outperform the other approaches.

Essentially, low-carb diets work because they enable you to become fat adapted. Insulin is brought under control and fat is burned as the primary fuel source. Our story subjects were able to shed weight and shake off ill health because they rewired their biological system to work efficiently – just as it was designed. Their systems are no longer overwhelmed by carbs and therefore constantly dysregulated by high insulin. LCHF turned them into fat-burning machines.

Exhibit A
Ebbeling & colleagues

Ready to look at some of the scientific evidence? Reading and understanding some of this is important, as it will help you answer some of your detractors, those people who (out of ignorance) still think fats are out and carbs are in. Ebbeling and colleagues (2012)[3] conducted a highly controlled metabolic ward study. Figure 1 (opposite) shows clearly that metabolic regulation and "energy out" significantly changed when eating the exact same number of calories, but from different sources. In this study, Ebbeling and colleagues helped obese subjects lose weight, and then put them on three diets for a month each. Everyone did every diet, one month on each, with participants randomly assigned to each diet. The diets were a low-fat diet, a low-GI (Mediterranean) diet, and an LCHF diet. Their findings support the hypothesis that dietary composition, not calories, drives metabolism.

The people on the LCHF diet ate the exact same number of calories, but expended a staggering extra 300 calories per day compared to those on the low-fat diet. This was measured accurately through a process known as direct calorimetry. That's equivalent to about 26 pounds of fat over a year. The LCHF diet made people burn more energy even when they were just sitting in a metabolic chamber all day with nowhere to go. You could call this increased

metabolism. And that's exactly what happened to Mary when she tried this approach.

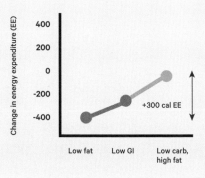

Figure 1: How the same people eating different diets containing the same amount of energy varied dramatically in energy expenditure.[3] The LCHF diet made people burn up more calories over the day.

There are now more than 40 randomized controlled trials (RCTs), which are considered the gold standard of scientific evidence, comparing LCHF diets to other dietary practices. I've put a list of recent RCTs [4-18] and review papers [19-31] in the references section for your information or follow-up if interested.

Mary's proof
—

"I went LCHF six months ago and so far I've lost 24 pounds. That was good, but what I learned about my body and food is amazing. Frankly, I'm happy, but I feel a little angry that it's taken my whole life to learn something so simple. Why wasn't I told about this earlier in my life? It would have been so much better. We've all been duped for so long, it's just a shocking situation when the whole health field got the message so wrong – at least for me. I lost weight effortlessly: I'm not hungry, I

have loads of energy and I'm off most of my medications now. All with eating more fat, not less."

Mary is still on the journey, but she has finally managed to get her weight under control by doing the exact opposite of what she thought was the right thing to stay healthy. More fat, less carbs, and her insulin is under control. "My secret is diligence, not effort," says Mary. "I have to be organized, I have to have the right food on hand. I have to be prepared. But I don't have to starve myself."

Exhibit B
The A to Z diet study

I've pulled out one trial to look at in more detail. It's the A to Z diet study, run by Dr. Christopher Gardner at Stanford Medical School.[8] Gardner compared four diets. There was a low-fat (in this case Ornish) diet, two forms of mixed Mediterranean-style diets (The Learn and The Zone), and an LCHF diet. More specifically, the LCHF diet was New Atkins, New You by LCHF advocates Jeff Volek and Stephen Phinney [32, 33]. I chose this one to look at for a few reasons. First, Dr. Gardner advocates for a low-fat, vegan dietary approach. Going into this research he was not a supporter of the LCHF diet. This is really important, as we all bring biases. Remember, the easiest person to fool is yourself. Gardner has done a good job at sticking to the data. Second, in this study, data is available to analyze from the individuals. This allows us to assess individual responses to diets, which is important because group averages tell us something about everybody, but nothing about each person. Third, they measured each person's insulin sensitivity, so we can see how insulin sensitivity affects weight loss. Fourth, he used "off the shelf" books to guide the practice. This is much more like reality than a study. So, what did they do and what happened? In Figure 2 (on the next page), each dot in each graph shows an individual percent weight loss (or gain) on each diet after a year. I've drawn those who lost some weight

and kept it off (benefit) in light blue, those who neither lost nor gained (neutral) in pale blue and those who gained weight (harm) in dark blue. This is a good way to look at what really happens in a scientific study. I have just included three of Gardner's four diets in Figure 2 (the LCHF, low fat, and one of his two Mediterranean diets, as the two Mediterranean diet results were very similar).

As an aside, it's important to note that no diet helps everyone lose weight. In some cases, people actually get fatter. That's the same in virtually every health and medical intervention. This becomes apparent when you look at drug studies and the variable "number needed to treat," or NNT. This is the number of people who need to take the drug for one person to benefit. NNTs can vary substantially: in the best cases with drugs like antibiotics, the NNT is six; in other words, for every six people treated with antibiotics, one will benefit. For drugs like statins that lower cholesterol, the NNT might be between 30 and 140, depending on the subjects and the study. Nothing has a 100 percent strike rate when it comes to health.

Looking at the four different diets, it becomes apparent that some people benefited from each approach. But more people benefited from LCHF and fewer people went backwards (gained weight).

More people benefit on LCHF than on other diets

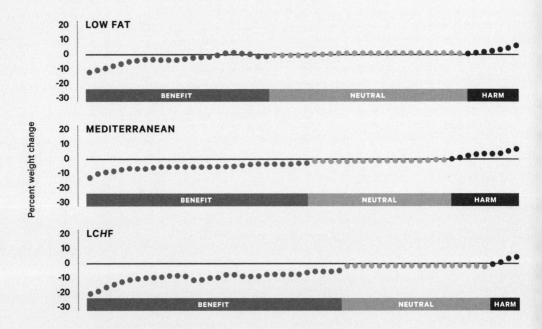

Figure 2: Some people lose, gain, or do nothing on weight-loss diets, regardless of the diet. On average, the low-carb diet has more losers, fewer gainers, and fewer people experiencing no change.[34]

Lawrence's proof
——

How did LCHF work out for Lawrence? We last met him when he was Big Lawrence at 18. He's just had his 21st birthday and he weighed in at 170 lb. He's gained muscle and is a good-looking young man. He's at university, doing very well. "I just went really low carb, but high fat. I thought, 'Screw it, I've tried everything else.' My mum gave me a low-carb diet book for Christmas a couple of years ago. It's a bit depressing when your mother gives you diet books, but I gave it a go and have never looked back. It's changed who I am. I'm not big, funny Lawrence who hides behind the persona.

I feel more like me." How did Lawrence do it? "I ate less than 35 g of carbs a day, kept my protein at moderate levels, and ate fat until I was full. That was that. In a year, I was in shape. I went to the gym. I put muscle on, and am now a lean 170 lb."

Lawrence is just one example. His experience echoes what we've seen in the literature, trial after trial. Yet the vested interests of scientists, the food industry, and of course the pharmaceutical industry, have kept us pursuing the least effective way to lose weight, keep it off long term, and improve health.

Exhibit C
Gardner & colleagues

Even more compelling is the data in Figure 3 (opposite). This time, Gardner and colleagues[34] show how an individual's insulin sensitivity affected the percent weight loss. What we see here is very important. Sure, some people lose weight on the low-fat approach, some don't. Those insulin-sensitive people do just fine. But if you are insulin resistant (those who actually need to get in shape the most), nothing happens on the low-fat diet. These are the people we often label as lazy and possessing no willpower. What this study says is that with all the willpower in the world, they'll still have a hard job of losing weight on these diets.

On LCHF, both insulin-resistant and non-insulin-resistant people lose weight. Everyone is a winner. Which approach would you choose if you were writing the national nutrition guidelines, or counseling someone needing or wanting to lose weight?

Diet outcomes vary by insulin sensitivity

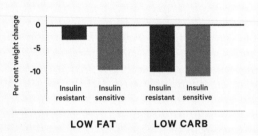

Figure 3: Weight loss is really only effective in low-fat diets if you are insulin sensitive. In the low-carb diets, it doesn't matter[34].

Leanne's proof
—

Lastly, remember Leanne? She got stuck in a low-carb diet after her husband had experienced some success. Initially, she was quite resistant. "Oh, I was annoyed with this stupid low-carb diet thing. Different meals (and everything) in a family is just hopeless. I decided I might as well join in and simplify the cooking regimen. Initially, I was just hungry and grumpy. I lost a few pounds and that was good because at least I wasn't putting weight on anymore. Subsequently, I haven't lost any more weight. I'm 145 lb, whereas I was 160 lb when I started. One forty-five is not what I weighed when I was an athlete, but I do understand I'm also not training twenty-five hours a week now.

"To me, the biggest surprise was how my sweet tooth dropped away. A while back, I was thinking, 'I deserve a treat.' I drove to the supermarket. I walked down the confectionery aisle. Nothing there interested me. I tried the cookies-and-cakes aisle, nothing there either. I tried the ice cream aisle, nope. I didn't fancy anything and just went home. It was a surreal experience for me. At no point in my life had I ever been able to resist these foods. I didn't crave them – sweets and chocolates – anymore. Wow."

The fat controller

This section is about understanding insulin and insulin resistance. We examine why Lawrence has been able to reset his metabolism completely and will likely be set for life. But how come Mary has plateaued? We also look at what else Leanne needs to change (other than food) to achieve optimal well-being. The differences come down to that master controller, insulin. Everyone changes constantly in how insulin resistant they are. The factors that affect this (stress, sleep, food, and genes) help us understand how to tailor our lifestyle (especially diet) to suit our individual needs.

The human fat-burning mode

Getting glucose into cells

The full understanding of how and why we get insulin resistant gives a "unifying theory" of modern disease, and insights on how to manage your brain and body to be the best you can be. That's why we want you to know all about it. When the body is properly regulated, the whole metabolic machine works perfectly. We produce insulin when we need to, become insulin resistant to help us when we are starving, and store extra energy when we are in times of plenty. In an evolutionary sense, this is a system designed to work across feast and famine.

Sometimes our cells find it harder to respond to insulin signaling. They need more insulin to do the job (that's insulin resistance), so they hyper-secrete insulin (produce loads). That sets off a metabolic cascade that can lead to diabetes, cancer, cardiovascular disease, and neurological issues.

Is insulin resistance bad?

No single thing causes insulin resistance, nor is being insulin resistant always a bad thing. Remember that becoming insulin resistant is a very important part of our biology. In our ancestral environment of feast and famine, we needed to become insulin resistant to store extra food as fat and to switch into a fat-burning mode to provide energy when threatened by starvation.

Insulin resistance without carbs isn't necessarily a problem. But in the long term, high levels of insulin (hyperinsulinemia) are very much a problem. This is caused by a combination of insulin resistance and a high-carb diet.

Mary's proof

Mary has been working away at keeping her weight off. You remember she lost quite a lot of weight quite quickly. But since then, she has plateaued. "I'm still doing exactly the same things food-wise, but I haven't lost any more weight. It's like something has happened and I've got stuck and can't go any further. I wonder why what has worked for me before has stopped working now. I feel like I could lose another 15 lb, but it just isn't happening, no matter how hard I try." Mary is what we typically see in a woman of this age with a long history of metabolic issues. She has been overweight almost all of her life. While she may now have her eating and diet under control, she has spent decades floundering. It's never been clear what her body will settle on as her ideal weight. Most probably, she is getting there now.

Would Mary like to be a little lighter again? No doubt the answer is a big yes, but it is what it is. She has success. She is feeling fabulous, looking good, and probably she might need to be happy with that. In the end, Mary is highly insulin resistant. She probably has a degree of long-term metabolic damage from having high insulin and high glucose her whole life. She won't get to a size 8 again, but she has already achieved success.

Lawrence's proof

No such trouble for Lawrence, though. He got down to 170 lb and successfully stayed there. "I've lost weight and now I can pretty much do what my friends do. I am fairly strict on staying low carb, but once in a while I drift off and eat whatever I want. I just carry on again." Lawrence still has a propensity to gain weight easily, and low-fat diets don't work for him because he is also highly insulin resistant. But he is young and doesn't have decades of metabolic dysregulation behind him like Mary. He was able to drop the weight and has kept it off. He has effectively reset his system. Sure, if he starts eating junk food, he will quickly shoot back up again. His lean (and always lean) friends will be able to tolerate more carbs than he ever will, but the occasional breakout won't harm him.

Insulin resistance + high carbs = big problem

A unifying theory of modern disease

Modern diseases such as diabetes, cancer, neurological issues like Alzheimer's, and cardiovascular disease all have multiple causes. But they also share a common metabolic pathway. Prolonged high insulin is the perpetrator. Hyperinsulinemia (see Figure 4, page 202) causes, or is at least associated with, almost all of what we call "chronic non-communicable" disease. Figure 4 illustrates the known scientific evidence for hyperinsulinemia and disease, showing how high insulin is implicated in causal pathways in virtually every major disease in modern society. Most of these diseases hardly existed at all until recent human history.

Outcomes of insulin overload

Figure 4: Prolonged high insulin is directly implicated (by good science) in damage to almost every organ and system in the body.[35]

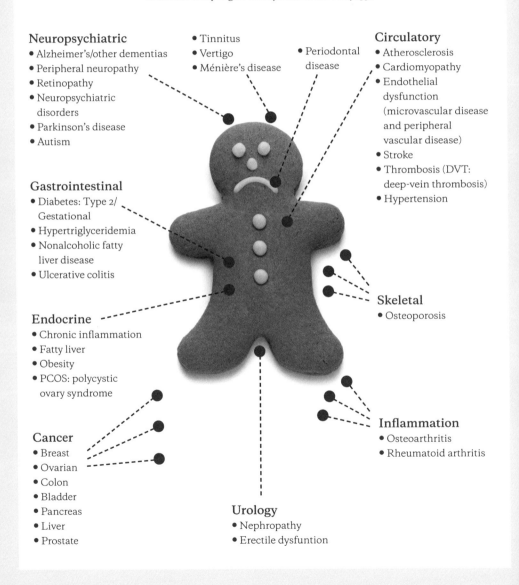

Neuropsychiatric
- Alzheimer's/other dementias
- Peripheral neuropathy
- Retinopathy
- Neuropsychiatric disorders
- Parkinson's disease
- Autism

- Tinnitus
- Vertigo
- Ménière's disease

- Periodontal disease

Circulatory
- Atherosclerosis
- Cardiomyopathy
- Endothelial dysfunction (microvascular disease and peripheral vascular disease)
- Stroke
- Thrombosis (DVT: deep-vein thrombosis)
- Hypertension

Gastrointestinal
- Diabetes: Type 2/ Gestational
- Hypertriglyceridemia
- Nonalcoholic fatty liver disease
- Ulcerative colitis

Endocrine
- Chronic inflammation
- Fatty liver
- Obesity
- PCOS: polycystic ovary syndrome

Skeletal
- Osteoporosis

Cancer
- Breast
- Ovarian
- Colon
- Bladder
- Pancreas
- Liver
- Prostate

Inflammation
- Osteoarthritis
- Rheumatoid arthritis

Urology
- Nephropathy
- Erectile dysfuntion

What makes you insulin resistant?

Insulin resistance is caused by a whole bundle of risk factors, most of which are "modern" problems. Some examples are stress that goes on for a very long time and insufficient sunlight. I've found 22 factors that could cause insulin resistance (see page 204, "The case against modern life").

Leanne's proof
—

Leanne's case illustrates the different causes of insulin resistance. She is the one who never really had a weight problem. She is essentially normal in her tolerance of carbs and not particularly prone to quick weight gain. For most of her life, she has got away with eating whatever amount of carbs she felt inclined to. This was especially the case when she was an athlete. Lots of carbs in, lots of carbs burned during hard exercise. She kept the scales balanced. What has given Leanne problems (and continues to do

so) is that she has multiple other lifestyle issues making her extra insulin resistant. Poor sleep, stress, alcohol, processed cooking oils, lack of exercise, and a whole lot of other things (see "The case against modern life" for the full list) are now conspiring to make her more insulin resistant. When Leanne is on holiday relaxing, these all disappear and she has much less trouble feeling good and staying in shape. However, in the day-to-day grind of coping with a busy family and a severely demanding work schedule, it's much tougher.

That, combined with a more difficult food environment (Leanne often doesn't have control over what is put under her nose at business lunches, on airplanes, and when she is rushing), means that she gets more carbs than she would choose on her own terms – and she gets them when she is stressed and therefore insulin resistant. That's a potent combination.

Insulin resistance + carbs + high stress = metabolic danger zone

Everyone changes constantly in terms of their insulin resistance. The factors that affect this – stress, sleep, food, and genes – help us understand how to tailor our lifestyle (especially diet) to suit our individual needs. Getting back to optimal health requires Leanne to address both her diet and her overall work stress. The key to understanding human health and well-being is understanding insulin resistance. When you understand the condition and what causes it, you can take steps to manage it.

Says Leanne: "Sometimes I feel like I deserve a wine, and that often leads to three or four. At the end of a stressful week, I might have had few alcohol-free days, missed most of my planned exercise, and be behind on sleep. I have also tried the very-low-carb end of LCHF

eating. But, frankly, with feeding a family, eating on the run, work lunches and travel, it is just not possible. Some people might have the organization and life to do this, but I don't."

Leanne's story makes it apparent that good metabolic health requires getting quite a few things right, many of which are really hard. Some you can't change – your genes, for example (see page 204, "The case against modern life"). But even when you can't get all of these right, an LCHF way of eating will help to reduce the damage. This in no way condones the unnatural modern stressful lifestyle. Optimal health requires all of us to take responsibility to get sufficient exercise and sunlight, and ensure we have a recovery strategy in place to prevent ongoing stress from accumulating.

The case against modern life

This section lists the 22 factors I have observed that contribute to making you metabolically dysregulated. Sadly, a system that was designed to cope with an entirely different living arrangement backfires against many aspects of modern life. These 22 factors highlight the reason why we vary so much as individuals in how much carbohydrate we can tolerate.

If you can return to a more traditional human lifestyle, it's likely you will be able to eat more carbohydrate without metabolic issues. This is because good health is about much more than just food. These other factors affect your health deeply, especially things such as stress, poor sleep, lack of sunlight, and pollution, as described on the following pages. These factors all affect your insulin resistance.

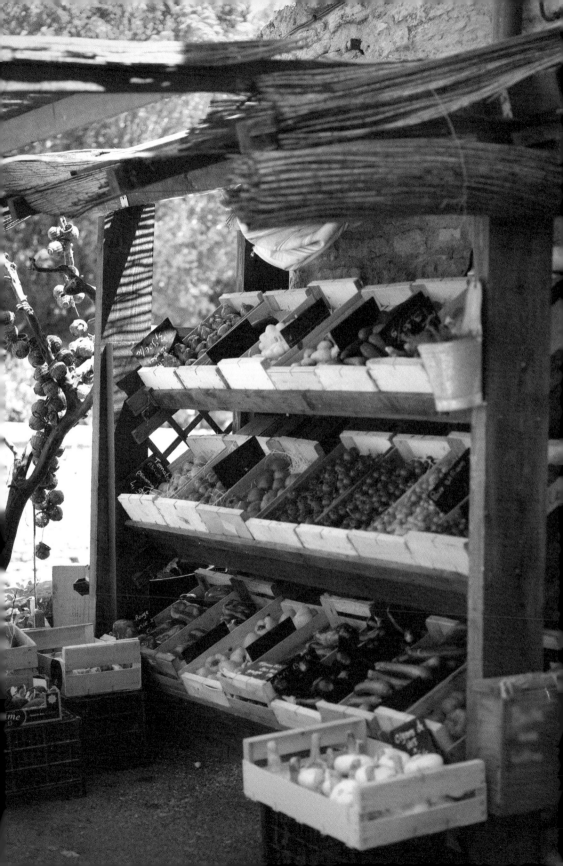

Factors that can make you insulin resistant

Factors that can make you insulin resistant	Probable mechanism and solution
Stress	Stress activates the hypothalamic-pituitary-adrenal axis (HPA) to release adrenalin and cortisol, among other measures to prepare the body for the "fight or flight" response (activation of the sympathetic nervous system). The stress response was designed to save your life, to go off quickly, even in the face of neutral or ambiguous situations. In modern life, this system can be switched on for days, weeks, months, or even years (known as chronic stress). The stress response was designed to be on only for a few minutes at a time. High stress with high carbs leads to insulin resistance, hyperinsulinemia, and metabolic dysregulation. That adds up to stress and carbs being a combination that will make you fat.
Poor sleep	Poor sleep activates the HPA axis, too. Same result as stress.[36] We are now sleeping less. We are less physically tired, less exposed to bright light during the day, and more exposed to "blue wavelength" light at night, which suppresses the hormone melatonin, which helps us sleep. Just think about how much better you feel when you follow the daily rhythm of light and dark to guide sleep - for example, if you are camping.
Smoking	Another message from Dr. Obvious. Smoking is bad for you. Smoking causes chronic inflammation, which makes you insulin resistant.
Not enough sunlight (low vitamin D)	There's good evidence that many of us are low in vitamin D - a hormone that helps regulate insulin sensitivity. Low vitamin D means insulin resistance.[37]
Too much sun (sunburn)	Vitamin D is manufactured by the body when exposed to natural light (UVB). Brief exposure to midday sunlight across plenty of skin will produce vitamin D. Vitamin D is also available from whole animals, including liver and cod liver-oil products. There's been a lot of talk about vitamin D supplements, and the evidence is best described as mixed. I said brief exposure to midday sunlight. Getting sunburned and having a deep tan will cause oxidative stress to your body, as well as inflammation. Both will probably make you insulin resistant and increase your risk for disease. Skin cancer kills.
Various pollutants and toxins (e.g., smog)	There is likely to be oxidative damage to cells and inflammation caused by a whole range of different pollutants and toxins, such as air pollution. This is a developing science.

Too much sitting	Too much unbroken sitting is an independent risk factor for poor health (meaning it's a risk factor even if you exercise). An enzyme called lipoprotein lipase (LPL) is up-regulated and makes you store more fat in fat cells, so you store more energy as fat.[38]
Lack of physical activity or exercise	Exercising increases insulin sensitivity. Exercise helps move and use glucose in cells. Lack of exercise does the opposite.[39]
Excessive exercise	Excessive exercise, especially when you can't recover properly from it, causes large amounts of reactive oxygen species (ROS) to accumulate in your body. These are inflammatory, they compromise immune-system function, and they activate the HPA stress axis. Excess exercise may also suppress androgens like testosterone, which increases insulin resistance.
Starvation	A lack of food means that your body switches to fat-burning mode. At least two types of cell – brain cells and red blood cells – don't need insulin for glucose uptake. The net result of starvation is that other cells in the body are temporarily insulin resistant so that glucose goes to the priority areas. This is exactly how the system was designed to operate.
High-sugar diet	Sugar is half glucose and half fructose, and does a triple whammy on the body.[40] Firstly, the glucose causes an insulin response. Secondly, the fructose doesn't cause an insulin response and mostly goes to the liver, where some is turned into triglycerides (fats). Some is stored as fat in the liver, and the remnants of the process cause insulin resistance through phosphorylation, uric acid, and reduced nitric oxide bioavailability. Finally, the more you go on with this state, the higher your blood sugar – which is itself damaging to the body.[41]
High omega-6/ omega-3 fatty acid ratio	It's likely that high amounts of omega-6 fatty acids (mainly from processed seed oils) and low amounts of omega-3 fatty acids (from things like oily fish) are inflammatory[42, 43] and cause insulin resistance. It's best to avoid the manufactured seed oils and eat more whole, actual food. Most people will be aware of the dangers of processed trans fats, which almost everyone agrees are unsafe. These are different from the naturally occurring trans fats in dairy products (conjugated linoleic acid or CLA).
Excessive carbohydrate load	When we eat more glucose (carbs) than our normal energy requirements, we involve the polyol pathway.[44] This means that a good amount of the glucose ends up getting converted into fructose, which causes more insulin resistance.
Time of the day	Insulin sensitivity in muscle follows a circadian (24-hour) rhythm. Healthy people are generally about 25 percent more insulin sensitive in the morning than in the afternoon or evening. So eating carbs in the morning has a different metabolic effect to the same carbs later in the day.[45]

High iron (hyperferritinemia)	Increased iron stores can predict the development of Type 2 diabetes. There is now a good working hypothesis that low serum ferritin is protective because high iron causes insulin resistance.[46] This is still developing science, but it's possible that eating too much lean muscle meat and discarding the other parts of the animal such as the fat, organs, and bones has resulted in high blood-iron levels for many people.
Various micronutrient deficiencies	Various other vitamin and mineral deficiencies are associated with diabetes and other chronic diseases. An aspect of this may be their involvement in glucose metabolism and cellular insulin sensitivity. This is one reason why we strongly advocate eating whole plants and animals with a low HI factor. If you are eating a range of these foods, there should be no reason for deficiencies or supplements.
High insulin itself	High insulin provokes a metabolic cycle that stimulates more beta cell growth and stress. Insulin is an inflammatory anabolic hormone. We need it, but excess is problematic. Note the vicious cycle - you eat loads of carbs, which raises insulin. This makes you insulin resistant eventually. Now even less carbs have the same effect, and so on. High insulin interferes with leptin signaling, making you keep eating when you shouldn't,[2] sending you further down a cycle of overeating and becoming more insulin resistant.
Menstrual cycle	Insulin sensitivity changes about 15-20 percent across the menstrual cycle. Peak insulin resistance is between 6 and 10 days after ovulation (starting at the early luteal phase). Increased insulin resistance is positively associated with levels of estradiol and progesterone, but negatively associated with follicle-stimulating hormone and sex hormone–binding globulin.[47]
Becoming pregnant	Pregnancy induces insulin resistance. There's a good reason for this - insulin resistance means that extra nutrients are preferentially shunted to the fetus and the mother relies on fat-burning.[47]
A fat tummy	Fat stored centrally (visceral adiposity) is especially dangerous for health, as it secretes inflammatory cytokines such as interleukin 6 and 8. These cause insulin resistance, among other problems.[48] For overweight men, storing fat around the breast area ("man boobs") can cause an increase in estrogen production, suppressing testosterone and causing metabolic problems.

Ethnicity/genes/ family history	There are individual genetic variations in how we respond to dietary carbohydrates. Some people are very intolerant to carbs, others less so. It's likely that this reflects exposure to dietary carbs and food security in people's genetic history. Groups like Pacific Island people are likely to be less tolerant of high-carb diets. Aside from other lifestyle factors featured in this table – and sugar – some healthy Asian groups can probably tolerate higher carbs.[49] Evidence from differences in genes such as AMY1 (the code for salivary amylase, the starch-digesting protein in saliva) shows some support for these differences. Groups with high AMY1 expression have a much better tolerance of dietary starch and a lower blood-glucose response than groups with low AMY1 expression. A recent study showed that people with high AMY1 gene expression were eight times less likely to be overweight or obese than those with low AMY1.[50]
Poor gut microbes	A field exploding on the scientific scene right now is looking at the billions of microbes that live in the gut.[51] Gut microbes affect intestinal permeability and inflammation in the body. This is part of insulin resistance. Exactly what constitutes good gut health and what affects gut permeability is not yet known. Here is what we do know: • Fermentation of plant fiber, seen in herbivores, also occurs in the human colon. Some animals (like cows) eat just grass and ferment that grass into fat, getting the majority of their energy from short-chain fatty acids (SCFAs). Cows on LCHF! Much of the fiber we humans digest turns into usable SCFAs. Some feeds the actual bacteria, some the gut wall, and some goes into the bloodstream and is processed from there. • The calorie count on products that contain fiber is flawed, and is another reason why a calorie is not a calorie. Celery is a good example of this: people claim that celery contains less energy than it takes to digest. In one sense this could be true – immediately available carbs are low. But you're not counting the fiber. If you do count it and then ferment the fiber into fat, you will end up with lots more calories. • High-carb diets that are high in fiber can turn into higher-fat diets, and that is likely what has been the case historically for humans. • Processed carbs bypass the entire mechanism and dump insulin-raising carbs into the system further upstream from the stomach and the small intestine. • Antibiotics are one way to destroy your gut microbes. Take them only when you really need to and make sure that when you do, you also eat yogurt with live bacteria in it to restore the good bugs in your gut. Tune in to this subject again as the science unfolds.

Clinical diagnostics for insulin resistance

The health system has some serious diagnostics that will indicate
if you are insulin resistant.

High fasting blood sugar

This is a standard test your doctor may order. You
will turn up to get blood taken in the morning after
no breakfast. Your doctor will want to see that after
an overnight fast your blood sugars return to
normal. If they don't return to normal, then you are
insulin resistant.

**HERE ARE THE LEVELS THAT SHOW YOU HAVE
AN ISSUE:**

- 6.1-6.9 mmol/L (110-125 mg/dL) – World Health
  Organization (WHO) criteria

- 5.6-6.9 mmol/L (100-125 mg/dL) – American
  Diabetes Association (ADA) criteria

High HbA1c

There's an even better way to measure how often your
blood sugar is normal. It's called glycated hemoglobin
(HbA1c). It shows the percentage of your red blood
cells that have been damaged by blood sugars.
Because your red blood cells are completely replaced
by your body every few weeks, your HbA1c level
indicates your average blood-glucose level over the
past few (probably 4-6) weeks. A normal HbA1c is
between 5.8 percent and 6.4 percent (40-47 mmol/
mol); higher than this means that your blood-glucose
levels are high at least some of the time.

Oral glucose-tolerance testing

This is a test your doctor will use to identify whether
you have Type 2 diabetes or prediabetes. It is usually
administered by your doctor as a standard drink of
75 g of pure glucose after you have fasted overnight,
and will show if you have high and prolonged levels
of blood glucose after consuming this.

A blood sugar level of 7.8-11.0 mmol/L (140-199
mg/dL) after two hours indicates prediabetes.

A blood sugar level over 11.0 mmol/L (199 mg/dL)
indicates diabetes.

What do the results mean?

These levels, by definition, indicate moderate to
severe insulin resistance, which has probably been
persistent for decades. If you have these, you will
likely respond very well to LCHF eating.

But it's not the end of the story. The problem is,
you can pass any one of these tests but still have
insulin resistance and all the problems described
above. Why? Because current medical testing looks
at our inability to get glucose into cells rather than at
how much insulin we are producing. Many people
can move glucose into their cells at an acceptable
rate, but need to use massive amounts of insulin to
do so. Herein lies the biggest unnoticed problem in
modern medicine: a large proportion of the population is told that they are metabolically healthy
when they are not. They take the tests and are sent
away being told all is well, and it is only when they
show "end stage" symptoms that we act. Do you see
the problem?

But can you observe symptoms yourself without a
clinical diagnosis? If you have at least four of the
symptoms listed on the next page, then it is likely
that you have insulin resistance.

Insulin resistance checklist

High and prolonged levels of insulin, even with a normal blood-glucose response, are dangerous to your health. Here is a (non-scientific) self-checklist for insulin resistance:

○ I've had trouble controlling my weight my whole life.

○ I have a large waist circumference (more than 39 inches for men; more than 33 inches for women).

○ I always feel hungry.

○ I often feel fatigued, exhausted, or depressed.

○ I have high blood pressure.

○ I have frequent hypoglycemia (low blood sugar).

If one of the glucose tests shows that you have high blood sugar, then irrespective of how you fare in the checklist you are insulin resistant. If you are insulin resistant, then carb restriction is the method that can best help you reset your metabolism.

The "carbohydrate tolerance" curve (Figure 5, below) illustrates that if you are very insulin resistant then you may benefit from being on a very-low-carb diet.

The carb-tolerance curve

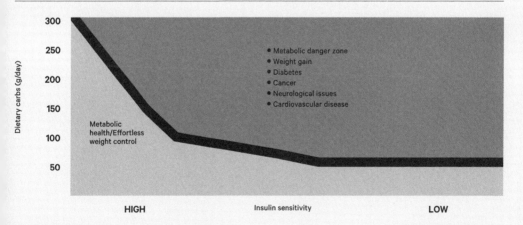

Figure 5: How much carbohydrate you choose to eat will depend on how insulin resistant you are. The left side of the curve is where your diet needs to be.

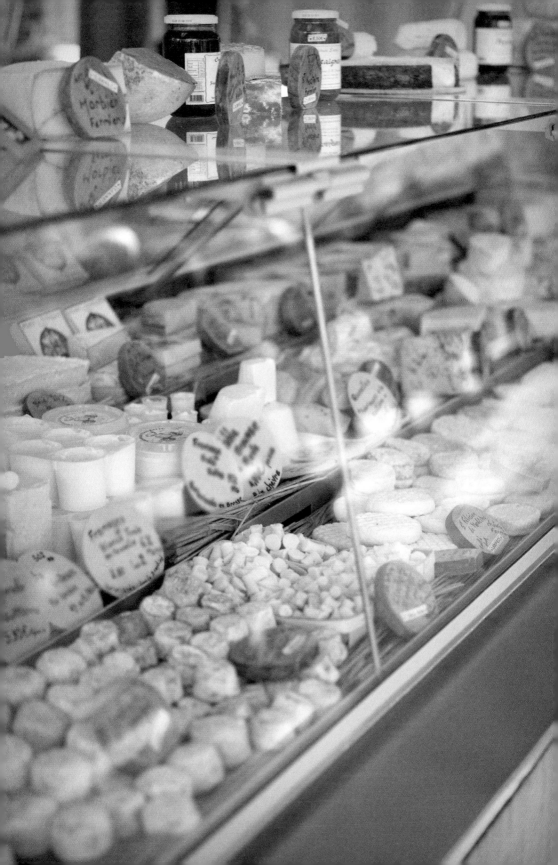

Eating fat doesn't make you unhealthy (or fat)

Fat phobia has led us to adopt diets of low-fat, highly processed, sugar-laden "fake" food.

In this section, we exonerate fat as the big baddie in health. To do this properly, we need to go into the scientific studies in some detail. How in-depth you want to go is your choice – remember, you can always go to the "WTF? The Science in a Nutshell" section (page 219) if the science becomes too arduous!

As already mentioned, insulin is the master hormone driving fat storage. Insulin production is driven mainly by dietary carbohydrate. While it is possible to get fat by overeating fat, this is hard to do in a practical sense for people eating the LCHF way. Your hunger and energy balance system is functional. Feeling full means that your "energy in" is better regulated.

Fat and traditional societies

Studies of traditional societies, both ancient and modern, show no evidence of harm from eating high amounts of fat in the context of a whole-food diet and a traditional lifestyle. The works of Weston A. Price (anthropologist and dentist)[52] and Vilhjalmur Stefansson (early Arctic explorer and ethnologist),[53] among others, make fascinating and informative reading. The fact that societies heavily reliant on fat have long histories of good health is the major breakthrough in understanding how dietary fat affects fats in the blood: it's not the fat by itself that leads to poor health.

Fats, especially saturated fats in your blood, are important to consider when it comes to your health. Saturated fat in your blood is associated with poor health outcomes, including diabetes, cardiovascular disease, and more. On the basis of "you are what you eat," it seems obvious to avoid eating dietary sources of saturated fats. But the body doesn't work in such an obvious and straightforward way: studies are now showing that different combinations of foods have a significant impact on blood fat. It's this subtlety that fundamentally undermines the traditional lipid hypothesis and informs our new understanding of why low-carb diets might be better for many of us.

Exhibit A
Forsythe, Phinney, et al

In a classic study by (among others) my friend, colleague, and the founder of modern-day low-carb research and practice, Dr. Steve Phinney,[13] participants were put on either an LCHF diet or the Heart Foundation's low-fat, high-carb diet (both of equal calories) for several weeks. They were fed meals resembling those diets and their blood fats were tested.

Even though the LCHF group ate three times more fat, and had three times more saturated fat in their food, their blood fats (see light-blue line in Figure 6, immediately below) were half that of those eating the low-fat, high-carb meals (see dark-blue line in Figure 6). This is called a deal-breaker where I come from. Eating carbs – not fat – translates into fat in the blood. Whoops, that's the science behind the lipid hypothesis proved wrong.

For the real eggheads, Figure 7 (below) shows extra data from the same study, but now specifically looking at saturated fatty acid (SFA) levels in the blood (left-hand graph). You see the same results, with the low-fat diet (dark blue) showing a poorer response than the low-carb, higher-fat diet (light blue). Cholesterol esters allow us to understand the fats in the liver, and demonstrate that low-fat diets have the same detrimental effect on the liver. Finally, if we look at changes in saturated fats produced by carbohydrates (a process called de novo lipogenesis), we see the same thing again in the blood and liver.[15] The fats are reduced by eating more fat and less carbs.

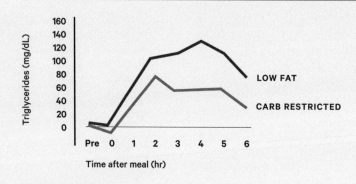

Figure 6: Eating carbs makes your blood fats go up way more than eating fat does![13]

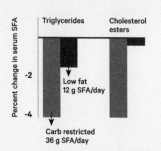
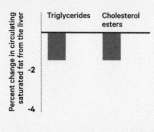

Figure 7: The liver fats go down less on a low-fat than a high-fat diet. The left-hand graph shows this because when you eat more fat, the blood fats go down more. There is evidence that the liver itself is producing some of this fat from the carbs: the right-hand graph shows decreases in saturated fats produced by the liver when you eat a high-fat but low-carb diet.[13, 15]

Exhibit B
The EPIC study

The final piece in the evidence puzzle comes from studies evaluating the impact of fat consumption on health over the long term. Big European studies, such as the EPIC study, which match people who develop diseases and/or die with people at baseline who were similar in all respects except for the fats in their blood (called a prospective case-control study) provide more specific evidence regarding the relationship between blood fat and health. The EPIC study involved collecting blood in 1993 from 340,234 people and following these people ever since. In a 2014 paper in *The Lancet Diabetes and Endocrinology*,[54] the authors identified 12,403 people with diabetes. They found that saturated fat in the blood, but not total fat in the blood, predicted diabetes.

They then looked at the specific types of saturated fat in the blood, and the findings got really interesting. It turns out that the length of the fat molecule, specifically the length of the carbon chain that is the "backbone," tells you where it came from (diet or otherwise). Even-chain fatty acids (those with an even-numbered carbon chain) can arrive in the blood from a limited number of dietary sources, but are also, significantly, de novo – made by the body from carbs – and the presence of these fatty acids predicted harm (diabetes). Odd-chain fatty acids and very-long-chain fatty acids come from dairy fats and both reduced the chance of diabetes.

The exact same thing was observed for a smaller group of the same people in a 2012 paper.[55] Figure 8 (below) shows that total fat in the blood is neutral and saturated fats in the blood are harmful. When those fats come from dairy we see a health benefit, but when they most likely are de novo (carbohydrate-generated) we see harm. This confirms that the lipid hypothesis is wrong and a more nuanced approach to dietary recommendations is required. So, yes, fats – at least saturated fats, but not total fats – in the blood affect your health. But it's how they get there that counts.

The number-one assumption of the lipid hypothesis is that eating fat, especially saturated fat, will make your "numbers" go bad, especially cholesterol. This is the most common thing we get asked about by those new to LCHF. But eating lots of fat, as you would in a low-carb diet, makes all the blood markers of health improve, including cholesterol profiles. High-quality randomized controlled clinical trials carrying out head-to-head comparisons of metabolic markers, including cholesterol, show just that.

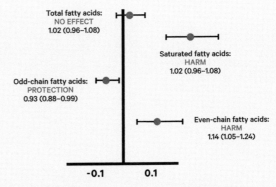

Figure 8: Saturated fat in the blood can still cause problems, but dietary fat probably isn't the problem. It's probable that fat made from carbs is more harmful.[55]

Total fatty acids:
NO EFFECT
1.02 (0.96–1.08)

Saturated fatty acids:
HARM
1.02 (0.96–1.08)

Odd-chain fatty acids:
PROTECTION
0.93 (0.88–0.99)

Even-chain fatty acids:
HARM
1.14 (1.05–1.24)

-0.1   0.1

Continuous odds ratio (95% CI) per standard deviation fatty acid increase

Exhibit C
Forsythe et al

I have chosen a study by Forsythe et al[14] to explain the impact on cholesterol markers; here, participants ate either an LCHF diet or a so-called "heart healthy" low-fat diet of equal calories. Forsythe and colleagues measured all the markers your doctor would collect, plus several more advanced ones. Figure 9 (below) shows how the LCHF dieters (light blue) fared compared with the low-fat dieters (dark blue). Note that improvement is indicated by a decrease (going down in value) in every marker except HDL cholesterol (which we want to increase). The study clearly demonstrates that the LCHF group showed better:

- Loss in weight (body mass) and abdominal (tummy) fat (ab fat)

- Improvements in blood fat (triglycerides, TG)

- Improvements in all of the modern cholesterol numbers we know to contribute to disease risk (see page 227 for the full explanation of cholesterol numbers)

- Improvements in all markers of blood-glucose control

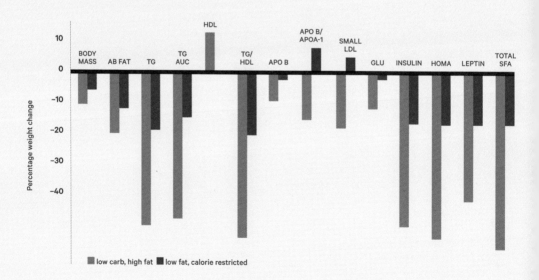

Figure 9: All of the markers of cardio-metabolic risk improve more with LCHF than with a low-fat diet.[14]

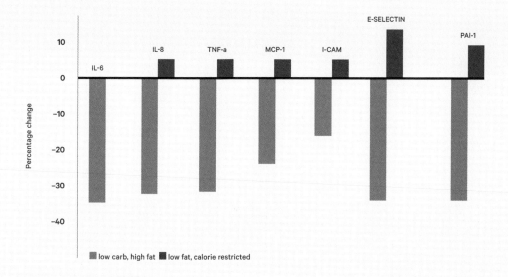

Figure 10: You can see improvement in markers of inflammation. Inflammation is thought to be a key determinant of poor health. The LCHF dieters showed an improvement in every marker of inflammation. The low-fat dieters showed at best no change, or possibly got worse from eating a low-fat diet[14].

Pardoning fat

The alarming truth is that fat has never actually been shown to be harmful. It's therefore arguable that the past three decades of fat phobia have caused more harm than good because the elimination of fats leads to their replacement with carbohydrates. Yet the health sector continues to endorse the food industry's low-fat slogans. The result has been a food supply that constitutes a huge range of low-fat, highly processed, sugar-laden "fake food."

Despite the lack of any evidence for what might seem like a reasonable starting hypothesis, the guidelines were developed. What's worse, after decades of no compelling or rigorous evidence supporting the "low fat" dietary recommendations, and plenty showing no harm from LCHF, public health continues to endorse the low-fat message. The biggest problem with low fat is that it also means high carb – you have to get your energy from somewhere.

What's more, despite evidence to the contrary, many scientists continue to describe full-fat dairy as harmful. They argue that we are living longer than ever (true), that coronary heart disease mortality and cancer mortality are down (again true). They regard this as proof that the simultaneous reductions in dietary fat and in saturated fat prove that fat and saturated fat are the bad guys. The problem with this argument is that it is based on correlational research. Correlation is very different from causation: correlation just means that there is a relationship between two things, in this case that

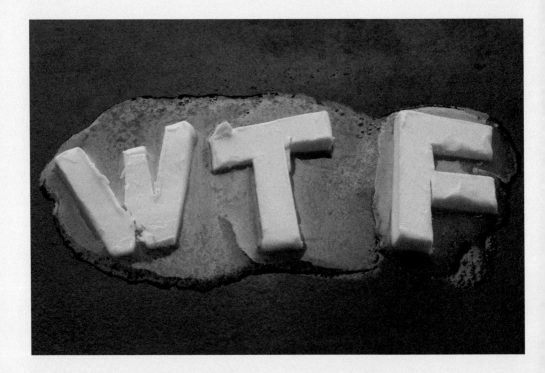

a period of reduced dietary-fat intake coincided with a period of reduced lifestyle diseases. But it does not mean that one caused the other, because there are so many other variables not taken into account in correlation research.

While it is true that we are indeed living longer, it is also true that the rates of disability before death caused by chronic disease are up. The modern trajectory is live long, die slowly – with lots of (expensive) medical care and a low quality of life. We call this high morbidity. Talk of reduced mortality rates hides the fact that many more people are living with disease. The reduction in mortality is more a reflection of better treatment than because we are eating less saturated fat. Much of the reduction in death due to cardiovascular disease is down to better care, prevention, treatment, and micronutrient availability (e.g., selenium in New Zealand).[56] The lipid hypothesis, with its public-health consequences (the low-fat, high-carb food pyramid), is plainly the biggest medical misadventure in human history. To be fair, though, we shall never really know the impact because the cross-sectional, associational evidence has no link to cause and effect. So my claim of medical misadventure is also only my hypothesis! What's good for the goose is good for the gander.

WTF? The science in a nutshell

Is LCHF safe?

If you've skipped the sciency bit to here, what you really need to know is that LCHF diets show at least short-term to medium-term improvements in everything we use to predict disease risk. That's good, and everything points in the right direction. The critics say that there is no long-term data on the possibility of harm. They say that there is no long-term evidence of safety. There are three reasons why the criticisms of LCHF are unfounded.

Evolutionary logic. We are proposing a way of eating that humans have safely eaten for most of the time we have been on the planet. You want long term? Well, it doesn't get much longer than evolution. Okay, the critics say that this evidence is useful in the puzzle, but not enough on its own.

There is no evidence of harm, only benefit (at least "non-inferiority," as we call it in medical research). Everything that current medical science considers important for health improves with LCHF eating.

We have a chronic disease problem in society. Our current dietary approaches are ineffective, and sometimes harmful. We see this in low-fat dietary trials such as the Women's Health Initiative, which cost $700 million and showed no benefit over baseline eating even with reductions in fat and saturated-fat intake, and showed harm to women with existing cardiovascular disease. [57] The view of the supporters of the low-fat status quo is that we need to do long-term studies which show that people can eat a low-carb diet for forty years without any harm being shown. This is absurd, because these studies cannot be done. Following their logic, no drug would ever have been approved, no dietary recommendations could ever be made, and most treatments in health, from psychology to smoking cessation, couldn't be discussed.

There is no way that a forty-year trial looking at a massive group of LCHF eaters will be conducted anytime soon. Firstly, it's just too expensive – it would cost hundreds of millions of dollars. Secondly, by what logic can we expect harm given what we already know? Is this sort of trial even ethical – especially running a control group for that length of time?

We need to understand that not embarking upon LCHF because it isn't backed by these trials is simply an unrealistic challenge when these types of trials will never get done. International evidence, and our own research, shows that the LCHF approach is the best option for people with insulin resistance and that it needs urgent recognition by mainstream health and medicine. No doubt nuances will emerge in the coming decades of research, and we will need to refine and improve practice. That is what happens in a young science like that of human nutrition. We need to start now, though. It's unethical not to.

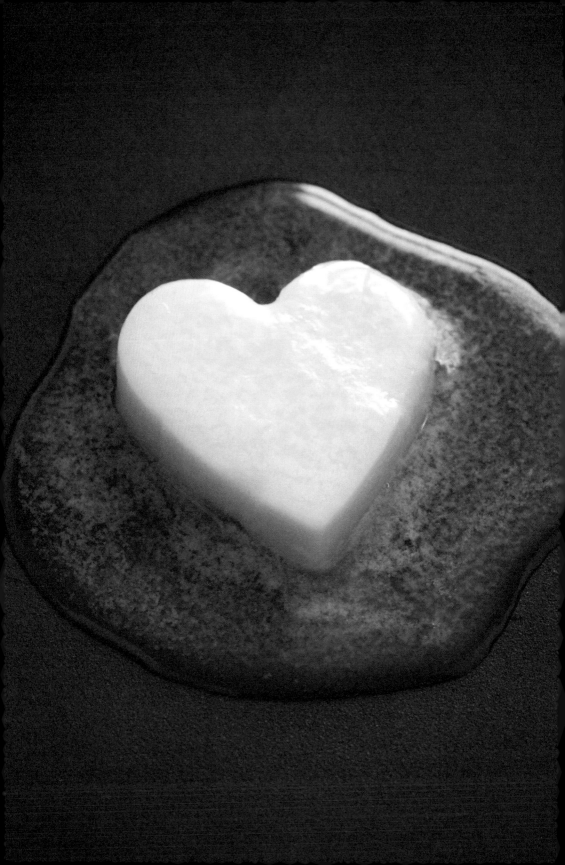

Is eating saturated fat safe?

Okay, so in the previous section we exonerated fat, but I know some of you still want to be really certain when it comes to saturated fat. Here, we dig a little deeper again with a focus on that alleged ultimate baddie – saturated fat.

Looking at the big picture (meta-analyses)

One scientific method for studying whether "X has an effect on Y" is to conduct meta-analyses. The meta-analyst will take all of the useful known data on the topic and analyze it again, collectively. There are specific mathematical techniques and rigor for doing these analyses. Because the debate about dietary fat, and especially saturated fat, has been so fierce, plenty of such work has been carried out.

A number of meta-analyses in recent years have found no significant association, in terms of study participants' relative risk of heart disease or total mortality, between those participants who eat the most and the least saturated fat.[58, 59] This indicates that the evidence linking saturated fat intake and heart disease is not strong. One meta-analysis, the Hooper et al study,[60] did show an effect of eating more polyunsaturated fat in reducing cardiovascular mortality when it substituted saturated fats for poly-unsaturated fats. However, the Kuopio heart study[61] showed that it was the addition of the polyunsaturated fat, not the removal of the saturated fat, that was beneficial – a finding also seen in a recent meta-analysis.[62] This is important: it is the addition of polyunsaturated fats, replacing either carbs or saturated fats, that provides a small health benefit for cardiovascular disease but nothing else.

Other than small possible effects on heart disease through this mechanism, there is no other evidence for the benefits of eating less fat, and less saturated fat. From the most comprehensive summary of the evidence we could find, intake of saturated fat was not associated with overall mortality.[60] Indeed, substituting saturated fat with polyunsaturated fat might make other things worse. The replacement of the ghee (clarified butter with 20 percent saturated fat) used in traditional Indian cooking with oils that are high in linoleic acid (an omega-6 polyunsaturated fat) and lower in saturated fat (5.6 percent) has been associated with rising rates of diabetes and heart disease in India. It has been suggested that this exacerbates an already imbalanced omega-6 to omega-3 ratio.[63]

Particularly interesting to us is emerging evidence linking high-fat dairy to improved health and low-fat dairy to worse health.[54, 64] None of these studies proves cause and effect, but they are at least contrary to what you'd expect if saturated fat, especially the dairy kind*, was harmful.

The burden of proof

I find it extraordinary that claims against saturated fat still persist given the lack of evidence of harm. The issue of dietary saturated fat and health is complex, and evokes very emotional reactions among scientists. But let's be very clear about one thing – in the context of a whole-food LCHF diet, there is no evidence of harm. In the context of the standard high-carb, high-fat diet (Standard American Diet), there could be issues, and these are likely to be due to unknown synergistic effects of fat and carbs together, especially in refined, highly processed foods.

Note from Caryn, the whole-food dietitian: Not everyone will do well on dairy. Some are intolerant to the lactose or the milk protein, and may experience symptoms such as bloating, gas, abdominal pain, and upset bowels. If that's you, then it's logical that you will have to avoid it.

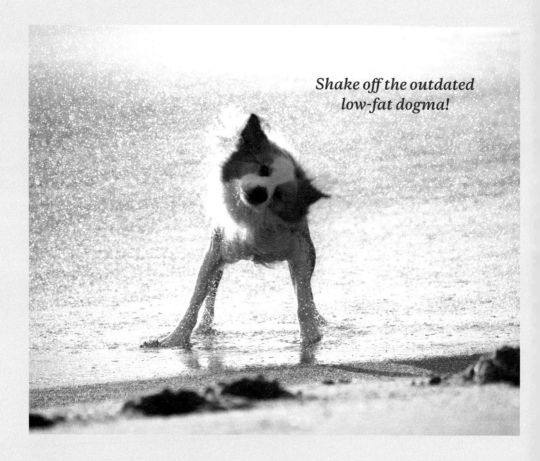

Shake off the outdated low-fat dogma!

WTF? The science in a nutshell

Is saturated fat safe?

Here's a summary of the actual evidence about saturated fat and your health, in plain English. This is really important, because before you embark on eating loads of fat, including saturated fat, you'll want to have some basis for your decision to eat more fat. You'd want to know that conventional nutritional thinking got it wrong. You'd want to understand what cholesterol is and what cholesterol numbers really mean. Here are the most important five points to know:

All of the combined evidence (meta-analyses) shows no effect of total fat on any actual real-world outcome, including death, heart disease, or other diseases.

Eating fat doesn't directly drive the biology to make you fat - carbs do that.

Eating both fat and carbs affects the fat in your blood, carbs more adversely than fat.

Eating lots of fat, as you would in a low-carb diet, makes all the blood markers of health improve, including cholesterol profiles.

But beware - the fat phobia runs deep. This is a major psychological stumbling block for many people. Eating more fat, which is a requirement with the LCHF lifestyle, causes psychological anxiety because we've been told for so long to avoid fat, especially saturated fat.

What about fats and cholesterol in your blood?

In this section, we look at Mary, Lawrence, and Leanne's blood results. They have all got thinner, but are they healthier? We learn what specific fats you should look at when you get a blood test, so that you are equipped to better understand your blood results. It makes sense to get your blood tested regularly when adopting the LCHF approach. It also demonstrates to anyone in your life who might be concerned about your increased fat intake that you are taking your health seriously and acting responsibly. Hard to argue with that!

The lipid hypothesis

The lipid hypothesis, also known as the diet-heart hypothesis, became popular with scientists, medicine (especially pharmaceutical companies), and policy makers through the 1960s and 1970s. A basic summary of those ideas follows.

Dietary fat is calorie dense. It has twice the number of calories (9 cal/g) as does protein (4 cal/g) and carbohydrate (4 cal/g). According to logic, eating fat is likely to make you fat.

The fat content of foods can affect the fat in your blood, especially saturated fats. Saturated fats raise LDL cholesterol (the so-called "bad cholesterol"). LDL cholesterol, and therefore by association saturated fat, have been conclusively shown to cause coronary heart disease. It is the LDL cholesterol that is the causal agent in the whole process. By implication, eating less saturated fat will definitely lower your risk of coronary-artery disease.

For years these arguments have guided nutrition and medicine, especially drug prescription. They underpin the (so-called) healthy low-fat food pyramid and subsequent variations, the healthy food plate in the US, and the national healthy eating guidelines of virtually every developed country.

The fats in your blood

Let's talk about the fats in your blood that you and your doctor will look at. Cholesterol is obtained by the body – either from eating it or from biosynthesis (making it in our bodies) – because it is an essential component of our cells' membranes. Cholesterol also helps in the development of hormones, vitamin D, and bile acids. It is essential for life. The way science has moved to understand cholesterol and what it does in the body has changed substantially over the past few decades. Frankly, modern medical practice is still catching up to the science. It is worth staying ahead of a rapidly changing field. Your health may depend on it.

Timeline of cholesterol research

According to my colleague and clinical pathologist in Melbourne, Professor Ken Sikaris, the science and pathology of looking at cholesterol has followed this timeline:

30 years ago

High cholesterol was thought to be a problem, while triglycerides were unimportant. It turns out that in some populations, low total cholesterol is actually a health risk.[65]

20 years ago

We understood that the two cholesterols that made up the total cholesterol (LDL-C and HDL-C) might have different effects. LDL-C was named "bad cholesterol," as it was associated with increased poor health, and HDL-C "good cholesterol" for the opposite reason.

- We now know that this is a simplistic picture: saturated fat increases both LDL-C and HDL-C, but has a differential effect on the size of the particles within LDL-C. Scientists also became aware that very-low-density LDL-C (VLDL) and oxidized LDL-C were likely to be markers of metabolic health.
- We also know that high levels of total cholesterol and LDL-C have been shown to be protective, not harmful, in some older populations.[66]

10 years ago

We developed a more nuanced understanding of LDL-C.

- The particle size of LDL-C can roughly be understood in terms of small dense particles (apolipoprotein B, or ApoB) that are potentially harmful to health, and large fluffy particles (apolipoprotein A, or ApoA) that are not thought to be part of the disease process.
- Trying to measure these in the blood requires an advanced biochemistry lab and is not standard (or even possible) in most pathology labs. While we know that it is better to measure ApoB and ApoA, we can't measure them easily so are stuck with the LDL-C and HDL-C numbers for now.

Today

We now understand that the combination of fasting triglycerides and HDL-C (both usually measured in your standard blood test) is a good measure of ApoA/ApoB levels.[67]

- Low triglycerides are correlated with less ApoB and more ApoA, so a low triglyceride level predicts a better profile. Higher HDL-C levels are also correlated with less ApoB and more ApoA. These two correlations are independent of each other, so combining the TG and HDL-C numbers together gives an even better picture. A good level for the TG/HDL-C ratio is less than 0.9 if measured in mmol/L, or less than 2.0 if measured in mg/dL.
- The actual number of LDL particles can now be measured by LDL-P (LDL particle number). Low LDL-P is a much stronger predictor of low health risk than low LDL-C, probably because the higher particle number means more chance of oxidation (oxidised LDL is bad). Low-carb diets reduce LDL-P, while high-carb diets increase it.

Take-home message for LCHF eaters

Low fasting triglycerides - less than 0.9 - means virtually no small, dense, harmful (ApoB) LDL particles. Good news! Eating a low-carb, healthy-fat, moderate-protein diet made up of predominantly whole foods will:

- Increase total cholesterol (TC), due to HDL cholesterol (HDL-C) and LDL cholesterol (LDL-C) rising. This is unlikely to be a problem unless you see very big numbers like TC > 10 mmol/L, which probably indicates a familial (genetic) high-cholesterol issue.
- Increase, decrease, or not affect LDL-C, due to VLDL breakdown - that's generally fine.
- Increase HDL-C, due to lower triglycerides - that's very good.
- Decrease the TC/HDL-C ratio. This ratio indicates the total number of LDL particles. As higher numbers are more likely to result in oxidized LDL which is atherogenic (which is bad), a decrease in TC/HDL-C is good.
- Decrease triglycerides (TG) and VLDL because of fat metabolism. Numbers below 1.0 mmol/L indicate a low number of small dense LDL particles - again, this is good.
- Decrease the TG/HDL-C ratio - a ratio of less than 2 is good.

What if really high cholesterol runs in your family?

There is a small group of people in the population who have familial hypercholesterolemia (meaning that high cholesterol runs in their family). This is typically evident among family members who have had heart attacks very early in life. For one reason or another, these people may not fare so well on LCHF, at least if it includes too much saturated fat. We don't currently know if it does them any harm in the long term to have massively high cholesterol numbers. But we don't know if LCHF is safe for these people either.

It's typical for this sort of person to have relatively high cholesterol - total cholesterol of 6-7 mmol/L (220-270 mg/dL). That number may go to 10 mmol/L or more on LCHF. Triglycerides can get worse, and

HDL is not that great either. If you are in this group, it pays to be cautious - consider eating less saturated fat. It might be okay, but we need more research here - that's for sure.

Saturated fat and carbs together?

It's plausible that eating too much saturated fat in the context of a high-carb diet could be harmful. There may be effects between sugar, refined carbs, and saturated fats that cause disease for some people. That's an extra reason why the Standard American Diet might be so harmful. I'm certainly not giving you a license to eat unlimited saturated fat. Rather, I am suggesting a diet low in carbs, high in fat: that's all types of fat - polyunsaturated, monounsaturated, and saturated - from whole plants and animals. In that context, LCHF isn't a high or unlimited-saturated-fat diet like our critics seem to think.

What the blood numbers mean

- **HDL cholesterol (HDL-C)** is often called "good cholesterol" because high levels of it are associated with a reduced risk of heart disease. Eating the LCHF way usually increases this healthy number.
- **LDL cholesterol (LDL-C)** is often called "bad cholesterol" because high levels of it are associated with an increased risk of heart disease. This number may increase, stay the same, or decrease when you eat low carb, but interpreting it requires you to take into account your triglycerides (see next bullet point). We know that LDL-C has two further sub-components: small, dense LDL and large, buoyant LDL. The small, dense particles are dangerous; the large, buoyant ones are not.
- **Triglycerides** are fats in your blood, and your doctor wants them measured fasting (when you haven't eaten for a few hours) because they are affected by what you eat. Triglycerides are most affected by the carbs you eat. That's right - the fats in your blood are driven by the sugars you eat! Low triglycerides (under 1.0 mmol/L) means virtually no dangerous, small, dense LDL particles. High triglycerides means that your LDL will contain more small, dense, dangerous particles with virtually no large, buoyant, harmless ones.

• **Blood glucose** refers to the amount of sugar in your blood. Your doctor wants to see the level when you are fasting because eating sugar means more sugar in your blood. This can be a bit variable – that's why you might also look at the next number, HbA1c.

• **HbA1c, or glycated hemoglobin** (sugar-damaged red blood cells), is a measure of your average blood sugar over the past several weeks. Sugary blood damages every part of your body, so you want this to be in the right range (see the next section).

The blood numbers you want

Before we have a look at Mary, Lawrence, and Leanne's blood results, here are a few key concepts.

Cholesterol is a waxy substance in the blood, essential for life but often thought to be involved in causing heart disease and other things if the levels are too high. This features as "total cholesterol" (TC) on your blood test. Total cholesterol is made up of two components: HDL-C ("good cholesterol") and LDL-C ("bad cholesterol"). Because of these two components, the total cholesterol measure is relatively meaningless by itself. Adding a good to a bad doesn't tell you much, especially under low-carb eating arrangements.

When you get your blood-test results, look for the following:

• High HDL-C (over 1 mmol/L)

• Low fasting triglycerides (under 1.5 mmol/L; preferably under 1.0 in the context of a low-carb diet)

• A low TG/HDL-C ratio (below 0.9 mmol/L or below 2 mg/dL)

• A low total cholesterol/HDL-C ratio (the lower the better)

• A low HbA1c (under 41 mmol/mol or 5.9 percent)

• Fasting blood glucose of preferably 5 mmol/L or under

• LDL-P (LDL particle number), if available, under 1000 nmol/L

Contrary to conventional medical belief, driven by the now-defunct lipid hypothesis, it's sugar and carbs in the diet that drive a poor metabolic profile – not saturated fat. See the full science behind all the numbers in the rest of this section.

What's up, Doc?

Mary, Lawrence, and Leanne have all had regular standard metabolic blood tests to keep an eye on things their doctors think might have a chance of affecting their health.

Mary's doctor

—

Mary's doctor was aghast when she first heard about her high-fat diet. Clearly what Mary was doing flew in the face of everything that was in the conventional nutrition guidelines. "She was really worried that eating all that fat would make me even fatter. And that the saturated fat would cause everything in my health to go terribly wrong. She encouraged me, no . . . she actually demanded, that I stop the madness.

"I asked her to keep a careful eye on my blood results and agreed that if anything went wrong, I would immediately reconsider what I was doing. After all, I was already on several medications and was a Type 2 diabetic. I didn't want to make things even worse than they already were."

Lawrence's doctor

—

Lawrence's doctor was already on board, as he was connected with a research center studying the effects of diets on blood fats. He was an expert in the field of LCHF eating, and in fact urged Lawrence to continue the regimen he had been so successful with. "He's a bit more open-minded with new knowledge in nutrition than most doctors, I guess. I'm lucky to see this guy from time to time."

Leanne's doctor

—

Leanne's doctor doesn't even know what plan she is following, but she does get regular blood tests. "I just don't really go to the doctor except with the kids. I don't have any serious health issues, so I just sometimes get asked to get a blood test to make sure I am on top of things. I probably only actually do the test once every two years because I never get around to the lab for the blood test."

Mary's results

- HDL-C up from 1.2 to 1.6 mmol/L
- Fasting triglycerides down from 3.6 to 0.8 mmol/L
- TG/HDL-C ratio down from 3.0 to 0.5
- HbA1c down from 55 to 43 mmol/mol
- Fasting blood glucose down from 6.8 to 5.6 mmol/L
- Total cholesterol up from 5.2 to 5.8 mmol/L
- LDL-C up from 4.0 to 4.1 mmol/L
- Medications: reduced dose of high-blood pressure tablets by two-thirds, ceased taking statin for high cholesterol, ceased taking insulin for diabetes (10 units/day)

———

Mary has made massive improvements in her blood profiles over a six-month period. She isn't perfect, but this is just an awesome result, one rarely seen using the conventional medical low-fat dietary treatment. "I've said this before, and I will say it again – I'm thrilled but also just a little annoyed it's taken me my whole life to learn these simple facts about nutrition and health."

Lawrence's results

- HDL-C up from 0.9 to 1.66 mmol/L
- Fasting triglycerides down from 1.7 to 1.0 mmol/L
- TG/HDL-C ratio down from 1.9 to 0.6
- Fasting blood glucose down from 6.1 to 4.9 mmol/L
- Fatty liver disease gone
- Psoriasis gone
- Better digestion and no more constipation, bowel movements 1–2 times per day now (was once every third day at some points on previous diets)
- More energy, and has gone from a student about to be kicked out of university to getting distinction

———

"My mum is more thrilled than anyone. I'm just a better, happier guy now."

Leanne's results

- HDL-C up from 0.8 to 1.8 mmol/L
- Fasting triglycerides down from 1.9 to 0.8 mmol/L
- TG/HDL-C ratio down from 2.4 to 0.4
- HbA1c still 39 mmol/mol
- Fasting blood glucose down from 5.1 to 4.8 mmol/L
- Total cholesterol up from 4.9 to 5.3 mmol/L
- LDL-C down from 4.1 to 3.5 mmol/L
- All traces of sugar cravings, desire for chocolate binges, and energy slumps gone

———

There's nothing remarkable here, but Leanne has seen substantial improvements in her energy levels, and some improvements in her blood fat markers – all while eating more fat.

Ketogenic diets and their therapeutic potential

Exciting new developments in science are suggesting that seriously restricting carbs so that the body runs on ketones rather than glucose may have positive outcomes for a number of conditions including cancer, acne, and neurological disorders.

In this section, we examine the next step on from LCHF - the ketogenic diet. Substantially restricting carbs pushes your body into a special state called nutritional ketosis. That typically means eating less than 40-50 g of carbs a day, depending on exercise levels and body size. At this point, your brain and most of your body will run on ketones, not glucose. Ketones create less oxidative stress and therefore less metabolic damage. Ketogenic diets therefore offer an exciting (and developing) new field of specific dietary therapy for some cancers, diabetes, neurological issues including Parkinson's, Alzheimer's and diseases of cognitive decline, acne, and polycystic ovary syndrome. We are far from knowing all the answers, and must be careful about prescribing LCHF as a cure-all, but evidence emerging from initial research and practice indicates the exciting potential of the ketogenic diet.

My thoughts on the ketogenic diet

In the state of nutritional ketosis, the brain and other organs predominantly receive their energy supply from ketones (beta-hydroxybutyrate and acetoacetate). Not everyone needs to be on a ketogenic diet. Everyone probably could be, at least for a while, as humans are designed to accommodate a low-carb nutritional environment with ease.

Some people go ketogenic because they prefer the way they feel energy-wise. Some choose it for therapeutic reasons. Others are motivated by the science indicating reduced oxidative stress and improved gene expression. Some, however, think that a permanent state of nutritional ketosis is inadvisable. It may, for instance, induce problems with thyroid function. Regularly moving in and out of nutritional ketosis is probably more likely to mimic the natural variations of food availability that humans evolved to cope with.

The ketogenic diet as a therapeutic diet

The ketogenic diet has been used, very successfully, for the treatment of epilepsy in children since the early 1920s. It is beyond the scope of this book to describe the ketogenic diet as a supplementary, or sole, medical therapy in other conditions. It is an emerging but incomplete science. We have already covered weight loss, cardiovascular risk, and diabetes (including Type 1 and Type 2) therapies in this book. If you have extra interest in Type 1 diabetes, I recommend you read Dr. Bernstein's *Diabetes Solution*. Ketogenic diets could be really helpful for a whole lot of things - we don't know the full answer yet. We have to be careful about seeing everything as a nail when you have a good hammer!

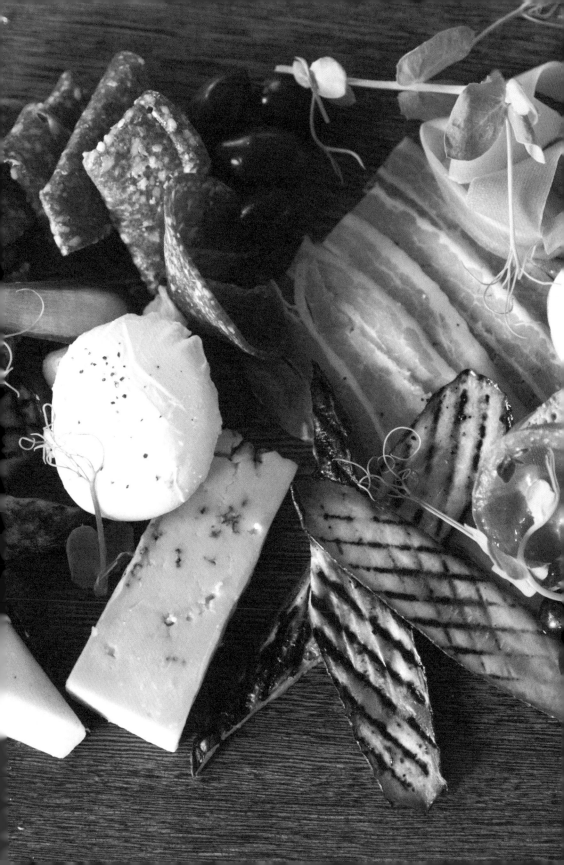

I am not advocating that you abandon conventional medical therapy that has been shown to be helpful (e.g., chemotherapy for cancer) in favor of diet alone. Consult your specialist and do your own reading (there is no excuse for not getting up to speed if you have a decent reading level and some basic biology).

Cancer

One of the more exciting areas in nutrition research and practice is the potential for ketogenic diets as an adjunct therapy for many types of cancer. The logic and research goes something like this: If a tumor is in some part of your body, that tumor will grow and may at some point metastasize. That means cancer cells floating around your body and starting new tumors in all sorts of places – lungs, liver, and brain. Not good. While diets high in insulin-raising carbohydrates might help these cancer cells to grow, ketogenic diets may provide just the conditions to reduce or even halt tumor-cell growth. Why? It has been proposed that using a ketogenic diet (that keeps insulin, insulin-like growth factor [IGF-1], and glucose low) stops the basic fueling mechanism for many tumors and is therefore helpful in getting into remission.

The evidence comes from several different lines. One is that diabetes is associated with high levels of cancer. Another is the Warburg effect (see below) – itself an established and important mechanism in the biology of cancer. Third is the therapeutic effect of ketone bodies on tumors that has been shown in animal studies. Last, there is a limited, but developing, body of evidence for the use of ketogenic diets in treating cancers (I highly recommend Fine and Feinman's review paper "Insulin, carbohydrate restriction, metabolic syndrome and cancer"[68] for further reading).

While we are not yet in a position to make definitive recommendations about ketogenic diets in cancer treatment, the future looks interesting.

The Warburg effect

The Warburg effect describes the peculiar mutation of most (but not all) cancer cells. Cancer cells can only use anaerobic glycolysis for energy. In other words, the cell relies 100 percent on the glucose fuel system. Without glucose, the cancer cell has no proper fuel source and can't divide – so the cancer can't grow.

This is really good, because what makes cancer cells so dangerous is their uncontrolled growth.

A second related mechanism, also part of the Warburg effect, is that high levels of insulin-like growth factor (IGF-1) stimulated by high levels of insulin further trigger uncontrolled cancer-cell growth.

If you get your glucose intake and therefore your insulin load down, that may be helpful because of the Warburg effect. The cancer cells are no longer stimulated, nor have the fuel for uncontrolled growth. The Warburg effect has been known about for decades, yet mainstream cancer therapy has taken little notice of it until the past few years.

Acne

There is some, although limited, clinical and physiological evidence that the ketogenic diet could be effective for reducing acne. Poor nutrition may cause the development of acne through stimulation of proliferative pathways. Foods under suspicion include those with a high-glycemic load and possibly some dairy products. Insulin production may be a causative factor in acne through stimulating insulin-like growth factor (IGF-1) and then a complex set of growth factor and hormonal biochemistry. People eating traditional whole-food diets – where there is almost always a low glycemic load – tend to have very little acne. Those eating processed Western diets tend to have high levels of acne. Severe acne is a problem, especially in teenage/early adulthood. I had acne and ended up on a drug called Roaccutane (isotretinoin) which delivers mega doses of a derivative of vitamin A. It's nasty and has horrible side-effects. If you or a relative suffer from acne, give LCHF a go. I certainly wish I'd known about nutritional ketosis back then.

Neurological disorders

Like cancer, there is an emerging potential for ketogenic diets to be therapeutic for a wide range of neurodegenerative disorders, from depression to Alzheimer's, dementia, and Parkinson's. Diet therapy has been attempted, successfully to an extent, for the following neurological issues: epilepsy, headache, neurotrauma, Alzheimer's disease, Parkinson's disease, sleep disorders, brain cancer, autism, pain, and multiple sclerosis.[69]

Why would a ketogenic diet have potential therapeutic uses across such a range of brain issues? By raising adenosine triphosphate (ATP) levels and reducing the production of reactive oxygen species in neurological tissues, ketone bodies have been shown to be neuroprotective. Normalization of abnormal energy metabolism in the brain may help ameliorate symptoms. This is not necessarily a cure for the condition, but its progression may be slowed. There is still a vast amount of research to be done in this promising area.

Polycystic ovary syndrome

Polycystic ovary syndrome (PCOS) is a common condition affecting about 10–30 percent of women. It mainly (but not exclusively) affects obese women. The primary problem is dysfunction of the ovaries. High levels of insulin increase the hormonal stimulation of the ovarian theca cells and interfere with normal ovulation. This makes pregnancy difficult. PCOS might also be described as hyperandrogenism.

The current "mainstream" treatments include those that reduce insulin resistance, such as exercise, diet, weight loss, and drugs such as thiazolidinediones or metformin (both are glucose sensitizers). Any intervention that improves (reduces) insulin and body weight may also be effective in treating PCOS. A ketogenic diet, in case studies at least, has been shown to be useful in treating PCOS. More research is needed.

WTF? The science in a nutshell

Is the ketogenic diet for me?

If you want to trial a ketogenic diet for its therapeutic potential, maintain conventional treatment under medical supervision and use the diet as an adjunct. Be your own experiment, and see what happens.

The ketogenic diet is now a proven therapy for drug-resistant epilepsy.[70]

Animal diet models show promise for treating Alzheimer's disease with a ketogenic diet. A few human studies show some promise, but much more work is required.

A few small clinical studies show that some people experience improvements in Parkinson's disease symptoms on a ketogenic diet.

Brain cancers may respond favorably to a ketogenic diet. I highly recommend that you look at the several excellent presentations online from Dr. Thomas Seyfried, a prominent researcher in the field.

Depression, migraine, amyotrophic lateral sclerosis (ALS), stroke recovery, and multiple sclerosis (MS) have case-study evidence and plausible mechanistic pathways for improvements. But all need more actual science of the costly rigorous kind for the medical world to take them seriously. Remember: absence of evidence may just mean that the work hasn't been done yet, not that the diet doesn't work. Again, stay tuned.

References

1 Pirozzo, S., et al. Advice on low-fat diets for obesity. *Cochrane Database of Systematic Reviews*, 2002. Issue 2, Art. No.: CD003640.

2 Saad, M.F., et al. Physiological insulinemia acutely modulates plasma leptin. *Diabetes*, 1998. 47(4): pp. 544-549.

3 Ebbeling, C.B., et al. Effects of dietary composition on energy expenditure during weight-loss maintenance. *Journal of the American Medical Association*, 2012. 307(24): pp. 2627-2634.

4 Adamsson, V., et al. Effects of a healthy Nordic diet on cardiovascular risk factors in hypercholesterolaemic subjects: a randomized controlled trial (NORDIET). *Journal of Internal Medicine*, 2011. 269(2): pp. 150-159.

5 Fabbrini, E., et al. Metabolic response to high-carbohydrate and low-carbohydrate meals in a nonhuman primate model. *American Journal of Physiology – Endocrinology & Metabolism*, 2013. 304(4): pp. E444-E451.

6 Tay, J., et al. Metabolic effects of weight loss on a very-low-carbohydrate diet compared with an isocaloric highcarbohydrate diet in abdominally obese subjects. *Journal of the American College of Cardiology*, 2008. 51(1): pp. 59-67.

7 Shai, I., et al. Weight loss with a low-carbohydrate, Mediterranean, or low-fat diet. *New England Journal of Medicine*, 2008. 359(3): pp. 229-241.

8 Gardner, C.D., et al. Comparison of the Atkins, Zone, Ornish, and LEARN diets for change in weight and related risk factors among overweight premenopausal women. *Journal of the American Medical Association*, 2007. 297(9): pp. 969-977.

9 Brehm, B.J. and D.A. D'Alessio. Weight loss and metabolic benefits with diets of varying fat and carbohydrate content: separating the

wheat from the chaff. *Nature Clinical Practice Endocrinology & Metabolism*, 2008. 4(3): pp. 140-146.

10 Brehm, B.J., et al. A randomized trial comparing a very low carbohydrate diet and a calorie-restricted low fat diet on body weight and cardiovascular risk factors in healthy women. *Journal of Clinical Endocrinology & Metabolism*, 2003. 88(4): pp. 1617-1623.

11 Samaha, F.F., et al. A low-carbohydrate as compared with a low-fat diet in severe obesity. *New England Journal of Medicine*, 2003. 348(21): pp. 2074-2081.

12 Volek, J.S. and R.D. Feinman. Carbohydrate restriction improves the features of metabolic syndrome. Metabolic syndrome may be defined by the response to carbohydrate restriction. *Nutrition & Metabolism*, 2005. 2(1): p. 31.

13 Forsythe, C., et al. Limited effect of dietary saturated fat on plasma saturated fat in the context of a low carbohydrate diet. *Lipids*, 2010. 45(10): pp. 947-962.

14 Forsythe, C., et al. Comparison of low fat and low carbohydrate diets on circulating fatty acid composition and markers of inflammation. *Lipids*, 2008. 43(1): pp. 65-77.

15 Volek, J.S., et al. Dietary carbohydrate restriction induces a unique metabolic state positively affecting atherogenic dyslipidemia, fatty acid partitioning, and metabolic syndrome. *Progress in Lipid Research*, 2008. 47(5): pp. 307-318.

16 Volek, J.S., et al. Comparison of a very low-carbohydrate and low-fat diet on fasting lipids, LDL subclasses, insulin resistance, and postprandial lipemic responses in overweight women. *Journal of the American College of Nutrition*, 2004. 23(2): pp. 177-184.

17 Yancy, Jr., W.S., et al. A randomized trial of a low-carbohydrate diet vs orlistat plus a low-fat diet for weight loss. *Archives of Internal Medicine*, 2010. 170(2): p. 136.

18 Dyson, P.A., Beatty, S., and D.R. Matthews. A low-carbohydrate diet is more effective in reducing body weight than healthy eating in both diabetic and non-diabetic subjects. *Diabetic Medicine*, 2007. 24(12): pp. 1430-1435.

19 Al-Sarraj, T., et al. Carbohydrate restriction, as a first-line dietary intervention, effectively reduces biomarkers of metabolic syndrome in Emirati adults. *Journal of Nutrition*, 2009. 139(9): pp. 1667-1676.

20 Boden, G. High- or low-carbohydrate diets: which is better for weight loss, insulin resistance, and fatty livers? *Gastroenterology*, 2009. 136(5): pp. 1490-1492.

21 Acheson, K.J. Carbohydrate for weight and metabolic control: where do we stand? *Nutrition*, 2010. 26(2): pp. 141-145.

22 Ajala, O., English, P., and J. Pinkney. Systematic review and meta-analysis of different dietary approaches to the management of Type 2 diabetes. *American Journal of Clinical Nutrition*, 2013. 97(3): pp. 505-516.

23 Dyson, P. A review of low and reduced carbohydrate diets and weight loss in Type 2 diabetes. *Journal of Human Nutrition & Dietetics*, 2008. 21(6): pp. 530-538.

24 Hite, A.H., Berkowitz, V.G., and K. Berkowitz. Low-carbohydrate diet review: shifting the paradigm. *Nutrition in Clinical Practice*, 2011. 26(3): pp. 300-308.

25 Kirk, J.K., et al. Restricted-carbohydrate diets in patients with Type 2 diabetes: a meta-analysis. *Journal of the American Dietetic Association*, 2008. 108(1): pp. 91-100.

26 Nordmann, A.J., et al. Effects of low-carbohydrate vs low-fat diets on weight loss and cardiovascular risk factors: a meta-analysis of randomized controlled trials. *Archives of Internal Medicine*, 2006. 166(3): pp. 285-293.

27 Paoli, A., et al. Beyond weight loss: a review of the therapeutic uses of very-low-carbohydrate (ketogenic) diets. *European Journal of Clinical Nutrition*, 2013. 67: pp. 789-796.

28 Schwingshackl, L. and G. Hoffmann. Comparison of the long-term effects of high-fat v. low-fat diet consumption on cardiometabolic risk factors in subjects with abnormal glucose metabolism: a systematic review and metaanalysis. *British Journal of Nutrition*, 2014. 111(12): pp. 2047-2058.

29 Seshadri, P. and I. Nayyar. Low carbohydrate diets for weight loss: historical and environmental perspective. *Indian Journal of Medical Research*, 2006. 123(6): pp. 739-747.

30 Sumithran, P. and J. Proietto. Ketogenic diets for weight loss: a review of their principles, safety and efficacy. *Obesity Research & Clinical Practice*, 2008. 2(1): pp. 1-13.

31 Wood, R.J. and M.L. Fernandez. Carbohydrate-restricted versus low-glycemic-index diets for the treatment of insulin resistance and metabolic syndrome. *Nutrition Reviews*, 2009. 67(3): pp. 179-183.

32 Volek, J. and S. Phinney. *The Art and Science of Low Carbohydrate Living*. 2011: Beyond Obesity LLC.

33 Volek, J. and S. Phinney. A new look at carbohydrate-restricted diets. *Nutrition Today*, 2013. 48(2): pp. E1-E7.

34 McClain, A.D., et al. Adherence to a low-fat vs. low-carbohydrate diet differs by insulin resistance status. *Diabetes, Obesity & Metabolism*, 2013. 15(1): pp. 87-90.

35 Crofts, C., Zinn, C., Wheldon, M., and Schofield, G. Hyperinsulinemia: a unifying theory of chronic disease? *Diabesity*, 2015. 1(4): pp. 34-43. doi: dx.doi.org/10.15562/diabesity.2015.19.

36 Novak, C.M. and J.A. Levine. Central neural and endocrine mechanisms of non-exercise activity thermogenesis and their potential impact on obesity. *Journal of Neuroendocrinology*, 2007. 19(12): pp. 923-940.

37 Holick, M.F. Vitamin D: importance in the prevention of cancers, Type 1 diabetes, heart disease, and osteoporosis. *American Journal of Clinical Nutrition*, 2004. 79(3): pp. 362-371.

38 Brown, W.J., Bauman, A., and N. Owen. Stand up, sit down, keep moving: turning circles in physical activity research? *British Journal of Sports Medicine*, 2009. 43(2): pp. 86-88.

39 DiPietro, L., et al. Exercise and improved insulin sensitivity in older women: evidence of the enduring benefits of higher intensity training. *Journal of Applied Physiology*, 2006. 100(1): pp. 142-149.

40 Akram, M. and A. Hamid. Mini review on fructose metabolism. *Obesity Research & Clinical Practice*, 2013. 7(2): pp. e89-e94.

41 Havel, P.J. Dietary fructose: implications for dysregulation of energy homeostasis and lipid/carbohydrate metabolism. *Nutrition Reviews*, 2005. 63(5): pp. 133-157.

42 Guldstrand, M. and C. Simberg. High-fat diets: healthy or unhealthy? *Clinical Science*, 2007. 113(10): pp. 397-399.

43 Bugianesi, E., McCullough, A.J., and G. Marchesini. Insulin resistance: a metabolic pathway to chronic liver disease. *Hepatology*, 2005. 42(5): pp. 987-1000.

44 Lanaspa, M.A., et al. Endogenous fructose production and metabolism in the liver contributes to the development of metabolic syndrome. *Nature Communications*, 2013. 4: 2434.

45 Jarrett, R.J., et al. Diurnal variation in oral glucose tolerance: blood sugar and plasma insulin levels morning, afternoon, and evening. *British Medical Journal*, 1972. 22(1): pp. 199-201.

46 Fernández-Real, J.M., López-Bermejo, A., and W. Ricart. Cross-talk between iron metabolism and diabetes. *Diabetes*, 2002. 51(8): pp. 2348-2354.

47 Street, W.W.H. Alteration of insulin sensitivity by sex hormones during the menstrual cycle. *Journal of Diabetes Investigation*, 2011. 2(4): pp. 258-259.

48 Esposito, K. and D. Giugliano. The metabolic syndrome and inflammation: association or causation? *Nutrition, Metabolism & Cardiovascular Diseases*, 2004. 14(5): pp. 228-232.

49 Wells, J.C.K. Ethnic variability in adiposity, thrifty phenotypes and cardiometabolic risk: addressing the full range of ethnicity, including those of mixed ethnicity. *Obesity Reviews*, 2012. 13 Suppl 2: pp. 14-29.

50 Falchi, M., et al. Low copy number of the salivary amylase gene predisposes to obesity. *Nature Genetics*, 2014. 46(5): pp. 492-497.

51 Fava, F., et al. The type and quantity of dietary fat and carbohydrate alter faecal microbiome and short-chain fatty acid excretion in a metabolic syndrome 'at-risk' population. *International Journal of Obesity*, 2013. 37(2): pp. 216-223.

52 Price, W.A. Nutrition and physical degeneration. A comparison of primitive and modern diets and their effects. 1939: Paul B. Hoeber, New York. Available at http://www.naturalhealingtools.com/articles/weston_a_price.pdf

53 Stefansson, V. *The Fat of the Land*. Enlarged edition of *Not By Bread Alone*. 1956: Macmillan, New York.

54 Forouhi, N.G., et al. Differences in the prospective association between individual plasma phospholipid saturated fatty acids and incident Type 2 diabetes: the EPIC-InterAct case-cohort study. *Lancet Diabetes & Endocrinology*, 2014. 2(10): pp. 810-818. Online: http://dx.doi.org/10.1016/S2213-8587(14)70146-9).

55 Khaw, K.T., et al. Plasma phospholipid fatty acid concentration and incident coronary heart disease in men and women: the EPIC-Norfolk prospective study. *PLOS Medicine*, 2012. p. e1001255.

56 Weickert, M.O. What dietary modification best improves insulin sensitivity and why? *Clinical Endocrinology*, 2012. 77(4): pp. 508-512.

57 Howard, B., et al. Low-fat dietary pattern and risk of cardiovascular disease: the Women's Health Initiative Randomized Controlled Dietary Modification Trial. *Journal of the American Medical Association*, 2006. 295(6): pp. 655-666.

58 Siri-Tarino, P.W., et al. Saturated fat, carbohydrate, and cardiovascular disease. *American Journal of Clinical Nutrition*, 2010. 91(3): pp. 502-509.

59 Siri-Tarino, P.W., et al. Meta-analysis of prospective cohort studies evaluating the association of saturated fat with cardiovascular disease. *American Journal of Clinical Nutrition*, 2010. 91(3): pp. 535-546.

60 Hooper, L., et al. Reduced or modified dietary fat for preventing cardiovascular disease. *Cochrane Database of Systematic Reviews*, 2012. 5: CD002137.

61 Virtanen, J.K., et al. Dietary fatty acids and risk of coronary heart disease in men. The Kuopio Ischemic Heart Disease Risk Factor Study. *Arteriosclerosis, Thrombosis, & Vascular Biology*, 2014. 34: pp. 2679-2687.

62 Farvid, M.S., et al. Dietary linoleic acid and risk of coronary heart disease: a systematic review and meta-analysis of prospective cohort studies. *Circulation*, 2014. 130(18): pp. 1568-1578.

63 Raheja, B.S., et al. Significance of the n-6/n-3 ratio for insulin action in diabetes. *Annals of the New York Academy of Sciences*, 1993. 683(1): pp. 258-271.

64 Kratz, M., Baars, T., and S. Guyenet. The relationship between high-fat dairy consumption and obesity, cardiovascular, and metabolic disease. *European Journal of Nutrition*, 2013. 52(1): pp. 1-24.

65 Nago, N., et al. Low cholesterol is associated with mortality from stroke, heart disease, and cancer: the Jichi Medical School Cohort Study. *Journal of Epidemiology*, 2011. 21(1): pp. 67-74.

66 Bathum, L., et al. Association of lipoprotein levels with mortality in subjects aged 50 + without previous diabetes or cardiovascular disease: a population-based register study. *Scandinavian Journal of Primary Health Care*, 2013. 31(3): pp. 172-180.

67 Maruyama C., Imamura K., and T. Teramoto. Assessment of LDL particle size by triglyceride/HDL-cholesterol ratio in non-diabetic, healthy subjects without prominent hyperlipidemia. *Journal of Athero-sclerosis and Thrombosis*, 2003. 10(3): pp. 186-191.

68 Fine, E.J. and R.D. Feinman. Insulin, carbohydrate restriction, metabolic syndrome and cancer. *Expert Review of Endocrinology & Metabolism*, 2014. 10(1): pp. 15-24.

69 Stafstrom, C.E. and J.M. Rho. The ketogenic diet as a treatment paradigm for diverse neurological disorders. *Frontiers in Pharmacology*, 2012. 3(59).

70 Katyal, N.G., et al. The ketogenic diet in refractory epilepsy: the experience of Children's Hospital of Pittsburgh. *Clinical Pediatrics*, 2000. 39(3): pp. 153-159.

Want to know more?

We firmly believe that individuals have a responsibility for their own health. Do your homework – there is plenty out there, both in the published science and in recent books. See an updated list of recommended reads and links at whatthefatbook.com.

OUR TOP 5 RECOMMENDED READS

Why We Get Fat: And What to Do About It, Gary Taubes (Anchor, 2011)

The Big Fat Surprise: Why Butter, Meat & Cheese Belong in a Healthy Diet, Nina Teicholz (Simon & Schuster, 2014)

The Art and Science of Low Carbohydrate Living: An Expert Guide to Making the Life-Saving Benefits of Carbohydrate Restriction Sustainable and Enjoyable, Stephen Phinney and Jeff Volek (Beyond Obesity LLC, 2011)

Fat Chance: The Bitter Truth About Sugar, Dr. Robert Lustig (Fourth Estate, 2014)

Death by Food Pyramid, Denise Minger (Primal Nutrition, 2014)

General Index

Recipe Index

About the authors

PROFESSOR GRANT SCHOFIELD

Professor Grant Schofield is leading the wave of change in how we think about our health, including how we exercise, how we sleep, how we (and our kids) play, and how we connect. The central role that real food plays in our health and well-being and a desire to help people "be the best they can be" drives his research and practice. Dubbed the "Fat Professor," he is at the forefront of challenging the widespread fat phobia that has pushed us to eat a diet full of processed, carb-laden food. "It's time to help the world change," he says. Professor Grant is a respected public-health academic with 20 years' experience and all the boxes ticked in a high-achieving career.

DR. CARYN ZINN

Dr. Caryn Zinn is a registered dietitian and sports nutritionist. Her master's degree was in the area of sports nutrition and her doctoral studies focused on how to achieve sustainable weight loss. Caryn currently combines academic work with her own clinical dietetic practice. She believes that this mix of academia and practice keeps her real and at the industry's cutting edge. "When LCHF first came onto my radar, I initially dismissed it," Caryn explains. "But going back over the evidence has convinced me that the current recommenda-tions are based on flawed science." Known as the "Whole-Food Dietitian," Caryn's mission is to influence the dietetic profession to understand the potential improved health benefits of LCHF nutrition.

CRAIG RODGER

Craig Rodger is a classically trained chef who spent eight years cooking in fine-dining restaurants, including Michelin-starred establishments in his native Scotland. Diagnosed with prediabetes at the age of 28 (an occupational hazard, Craig says, for chefs tasting the highly refined cuisine designed to pleasure discerning gourmands), he felt compelled to research and adopt a different approach to eating and cooking. Craig and his family are the founders of LOOP, New Zealand's first restaurant to feature an LCHF approach to dining out. Craig has a real passion for stripping away carb-laden fillers and for using nutritionally dense ingredients as the foundation of culinary excellence. He is no longer prediabetic.

Contributors

PETE EVANS

Pete Evans is a chef, health coach, television presenter, and best-selling author with more than 10 cookbooks to his name, including *Healthy Every Day*, *The Paleo Chef*, and *Going Paleo*. He is passionate about sharing the LCHF message and changing the lives of people around him.

NINA TEICHOLZ

Nina Teicholz is a science journalist and author of the *The Big Fat Surprise*, an international and *New York Times* best seller that has upended the conventional wisdom on dietary fat, especially saturated fat. She is a leader in current efforts to ensure that national nutrition policies are evidence based.

Acknowledgments

Writing *What the Fat?* has been an enormous project, relying on help from all sorts of committed and generous people. Special thanks go to Helen Kilding, Dr Katie Robinson, and George Henderson, who have all provided valuable content feedback that has helped this book be what it is.

We also thank Catherine Crofts, Dr. Simon Thornley, Kate White, Dee Holdsworth Perks, Dr. Lisa Mackay, Hannah Gerdin, Jo Dickson, Anne Schofield, the Sopers - Liz and Gordon, Brodwyn Boock, Chefs Garry Trewin and Louis Nieuwenhujsen, Peta Laery, Kerry Dunphy, Jane Mackenzie, Sally Rowe, and Brydie Harris, who have all provided feedback and help to us at one time or another along this book's journey. We listened carefully to everything you had to say. Associate Professor Geoff Dickson and Dee Parry, you both provided some editing and proofing for us, but most of all you delivered on the creativity for the book.

Thanks to Cindy, Trish, Gary, Helen, Mary, Lawrence, Leanne, and Sheree, our friends and clients who provided us with testimonials to bring the LCHF story to life.

And finally to our supportive and long-suffering partners, Dr. Louise Schofield, Mark Dawson, and Hailey Rodger. We know the bigger part you have all played in this project and beyond; joining us in our challenge to conventional and outdated wisdom in nutrition. We thank you so much for everything - enabling us to go further, in our mission to change the world, than we would ever have been capable of on our own.

Follow us
whatthefatbook.com
facebook.com/whatthefatbook
twitter.com/whatthefatbook

Professor Grant Schofield
profgrant.com
twitter.com/grantsnz

Dr. Caryn Zinn
carynzinn.com
facebook.com/carynzinndietitian
twitter.com/carynzinn

Craig Rodger
facebook.com/chefcraigrodger
twitter.com/chefcraigwtf

weldon**owen**

Published in North America by Weldon Owen
1045 Sansome Street, San Francisco, CA 94111
www.weldonowen.com
Weldon Owen is a division of Bonnier Publishing USA

Photography: Scottie T Photography, except where
outlined below
Additional images by: Cameron Gibb pages 58 (right), 105,
106, 111, 118 (bottom right), 120, 123, 125, 127, 139, 141, 156,
157, 171, 173; Geoff Blackwell page 63; iStock pages 132, 153,
155, 170, 172, 175, 202, 220, front cover; Getty Images back cover;
Rachael McKenna pages 181, 205, 212

ISBN 978-1-68188-230-7

Library of Congress Cataloging-in-Publication data is available

Printed and bound in China

This edition printed in 2017
10 9 8 7 6 5 4 3 2 1